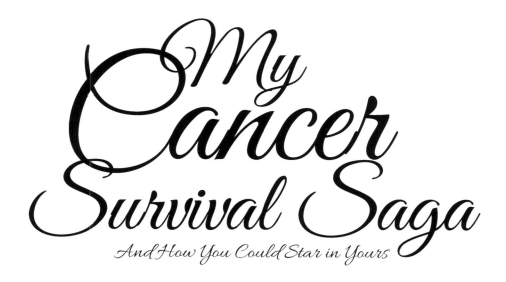

My Cancer Survival Saga

And How You Could Star in Yours

Jen Kimberley

BALBOA.PRESS

A DIVISION OF HAY HOUSE

Balboa Press books may be ordered through booksellers or by contacting:

Balboa Press
A Division of Hay House
1663 Liberty Drive
Bloomington, IN 47403
www.balboapress.com.au
AU TFN: 1 800 844 925 (Toll Free inside Australia)
AU Local: 0283 107 086 (+61 2 8310 7086 from outside Australia)

Because of the dynamic nature of the Internet, any web addresses or links contained in this book may have changed since publication and may no longer be valid. The views expressed in this work are solely those of the author and do not necessarily reflect the views of the publisher, and the publisher hereby disclaims any responsibility for them.

The author of this book does not dispense medical advice or prescribe the use of any technique as a form of treatment for physical, emotional, or medical problems without the advice of a physician, either directly or indirectly. The intent of the author is only to offer information of a general nature to help you in your quest for emotional and spiritual well-being. In the event you use any of the information in this book for yourself, which is your constitutional right, the author and the publisher assume no responsibility for your actions.

The information, ideas, and suggestions in this book are not intended as a substitute for professional medical advice. Before following any suggestions contained in this book, you should consult your personal physician. Neither the author nor the publisher shall be liable or responsible for any loss or damage allegedly arising as a consequence of your use or application of any information or suggestions in this book.

Any people depicted in stock imagery provided by Thinkstock are models, and such images are being used for illustrative purposes only. Certain stock imagery © Thinkstock.

Print information available on the last page.

ISBN: 978-1-5043-0371-2 (sc)
ISBN: 978-1-5043-0372-9 (e)

Balboa Press rev. date: 10/07/2020

"Employ your time in improving yourself by other men's writings, so that you shall gain easily what others have labored hard for."

--- Socrates

Table of Contents

Table of Sidebars

Table of Graphics

Acknowledgements

Very deep thanks to Dr. Thomas Lodi and his clinic staff in Arizona for getting me through the severe leukemia acute phase and for providing access to stem cell treatments in Thailand.

Very deep thanks also to Dr. Henning Saupe and his clinic staff in Germany for waking my immune system up, tolerating my erratic behavior, and doing some much-needed testing.

Very warm thanks to my best High School friend, Margaret Kennedy, for reviewing this whole Saga and sending me her response. We had so many great bike rides together on the country roads around Armidale, N.S.W. As she said recently, remembering those days, "The wind in your hair and a mate by your side! Great memories!"

Many thanks also to Bill Henderson, RIP. He was 84 and a much-loved teacher in the alternative cancer treatment world. I was one of the many cancer patients who used his protocol and received his coaching.

And of course, enormous loving thanks to my son Dmitri Kalmar, who gave his long-awaited vacation time to his mother in her dire need. There would be no Saga if he had not brought me from Costa Rica to Arizona and stayed to get me settled and equipped and well-cared-for.

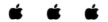

This book is dedicated to my son, Dmitri George Kalmar,
computer programmer extraordinaire,
who saved my life when I had a cancer-caused stroke
in a foreign country and was helpless.
He is the most caring son
any mother could wish for.

Preface

In this Saga, I've used a concise style. No throat clearing. No saying what you're going to say, then saying it, then saying what you've just said. There are two voices: the main narrative is a conversational style and the separated text uses an objective style giving facts about something.

This is not a compendium of alternative cancer treatments; there are other such books available already. It's my personal story with ancilliary neutral information. I have had leukemia for 18 years and the narrative tells the story of why it's been so long, what treatments I've had in the alternative cancer world, and how come I'm still running around when I was supposed to bow out eight years ago. It describes mistakes I made and things I learned the hard way and people who helped me. If you want to know more about cancer treatments other than the three conventional ones of chemotherapy, radiation and surgery, this book is for you. And if you want to know how it feels to receive those alternative treatments, ditto. Please read on.

This Saga also offers five sections on aspects of energy work and how to start clearing, validating and protecting your own space. Here and there it contains humor, something that tends to disappear when you get the "big C" diagnosis but which is highly valuable for recovery. If you are a cancer patient, I hope this book gives you some companionship, some friendly company along the cancer road, which can be a lonely and difficult trek.

For ongoing information and ideas, please see www.jenkimberley.com. I hope this Saga is helpful for you and if you have cancer you have my strong good wishes for a successful recovery.

Jen Kimberley,

Carbondale, Illinois,

December, 2019

Introduction

Although being handed a cancer diagnosis can be alarming, even terrifying, it does have a positive side. It's a form of feedback from Life or from planet Earth. Feedback, whether positive or negative, is at least new information or a new point of view and most of us tend to get stuck in certain outlooks and lifestyles, forgetting that there are many others just as valid as ours. A cancer diagnosis is a wake-up call if you like. It's Life tapping you on the shoulder and saying, "Watch your step, there's a cliff up ahead".

The predominant treatment approach views cancer as an enemy and both taxpayer money and private donations have been funding the War on Cancer since 1971. In this long war, just three weapons make up the arsenal:

1. Surgery;

2. Radiation; and

3. Chemotherapy.

These weapons can reduce or eliminate tumors and put a patient "in remission". That remission may last several years until the cancer returns. And if those three weapons fail to help, the patient may hear:

"I'm sorry, but we can do nothing more for you. I suggest you go home and make sure your affairs are in order."

For an anxious recipient of the Big C Diagnosis, it does not help to regard cancer as an enemy that must be fought to the bitter end; as an implacable foe that must be defeated; as something outside ourselves that attacked us. Living in fear and antagonism is counter to good health.

Everyone has cancer cells. They form constantly and if your immune system is in good repair, it constantly disposes of them. There's good balance there and good health is all about good balance. If cancer cells build up faster than one's system can vanquish them, Cancer develops until it becomes big enough to be detected by a medical test. By the time one receives the diagnosis, Cancer has likely been growing in the body for months or years. It might have given you symptoms such as fatigue, headaches, obscure aches and pains, or digestive problems, but nobody knew what caused those things so you just picked up something from the drug store and moved on.

Cause and Cure: A Partnership

The treatment model of "kill cancer cells" is like one hand trying to clap. Consider a healthy body's natural balance between cancer cell formation and immune system disposal of those cells. Surely that provides a good treatment model:

- Dispose of cancer cells and simultaneously increase immune system strength. Two hands clapping.

Has your cancer doctor asked you about your eating habits? Have you been given any tests to determine your body's acidity or alkalinity, oxygen saturation levels, colon health, presence of parasites, nutritional deficiencies or overloads, or food allergies (sensitivities)? There are various theories as to cancer causation (see Chapter 10) and medical tradition favors the genetic theory, that cancer is caused by genetic factors that cannot be changed. If the cause is fixed in place, no cure is possible and changing a patient's diet or pH levels and so forth would be pointless. Most conventional cancer doctors see no reason to address the above issues.

The causation theory that lies beneath this Saga is the lifestyle theory. That theory also lies beneath the work of many alternative or integrative cancer clinics and the work of many doctors and naturopaths. We now have many more health options than our parents and grandparents did. With some online searching, we can find numerous medical professionals, eager to share their knowledge and experience with us and show us how to effectively deal with cancer. So the question becomes: How do we choose among them?

Testing, Customizing and Detoxifying

Your cancer is not just "a case of colon cancer" or "another case of breast cancer". It's your particular bodily disarray and malfunction, caused by the specific conditions in your body that you were either born with or have developed over the years.

Nor is the disarray just your particular combination of things that shouldn't be in any human body – it's also the things missing that should be there. Years of junk food leave a person malnourished. And poor soil from destructive agriculture practices stocks the supermarket with foods that may look the same as they did to our grandparents but no longer contain the nutrients they once did.

For most of us, cancer is like a large jigsaw puzzle and the box has no picture to guide you in assembling it. We spread the pieces on a table and get a quick impression of colors; we pick out the edge and corner pieces and get them fitted together; then what? To implement successful healing (solve the puzzle), we first must have a model or image to guide us, a specific goal or set of goals to aim for. We tend to take our body functions for granted – digestion, breathing, excretion, healing of minor injuries etc. But a Cancer diagnosis tells us that something is not working right. Probably many things.

It tells us that our body cells are **deficient in oxygen** for whatever reason and that our **body pH is too acidic**. It may also be telling us that we are not absorbing all the nutrients we eat; or our colon is not letting go of all the toxic matter headed for the exit; or some stuck emotions are interfering with our body's energy flow. Or other things.

Caveat: The lifestyle causation theory pinpoints dietary and lifestyle habits but it would not really be fair to say that it's our fault we got cancer. One might see that as theoretically true, but in practice, we were living our lives the best we could, busy with dozens of concerns, problems and projects, and didn't know that cancer cells were becoming too numerous. Once we start learning that, however, and seeing all our options, I think it would be fair to say it's our responsibility to take the best action we can. The upside of the lifestyle theory is that it gives us control over our own health.

1. Testing

How do we start building a puzzle guidance picture? First, by learning more about the body's general ill-health. A well body will not develop cancer. Listening to your body, paying attention to its little messages such as headaches at certain times, assorted skin problems, or chronic digestive discomfort will help you know what to investigate, thus what tests to start with.

We can choose from a plethora of laboratory tests – food allergies, vitamin and mineral levels in the body, a Candida test, leaky gut test, heavy metal test, blood tests, stool tests, urine tests – your doctor or naturopath can order these for

> It is far more important to know what person the disease has than what disease the person has.
>
> ---Hippocrates, 460 to 377 B.C.

you and discuss the results with you. These results will no doubt suggest further testing to clarify issues and answer questions. As the results of each test give you bits of information, you can gradually build a clear picture of your ill-health and thus know what conditions to correct. For more on testing, please see Chapter 7.

2. **Customizing**

Nobody else's cancer is exactly like yours. Nobody else has the exact genetic make-up that you have and not even identical twins are duplicates of each other because two different spirits are living in the two bodies, making different decisions, following different life-paths. When we start to understand our overall ill-health, we can start removing its causes rather than continually buying remedies that do only symptom suppression.

When looking at cancer protocols, I would suggest that you don't try a bit of this and some of that and buy this equipment or that. A hodge-podge won't work. On the internet, many of the doctors, naturopaths, and other medical practitioners offering cancer treatments, theories, and warnings also sell products to address this or that problem. They all spring from tremendous amounts of knowledge and experience and I'd say the products (supplements or treatment devices) tend to be of superior quality. But in most cases, these are "one cure fits all" offerings.

And we need to keep in mind that any person selling something online, including space in a cancer clinic, has somewhat different priorities than we do as cancer patients. They are making a living; we are sick and need exactly the right treatment(s) to get well. Treatments we can afford. Alternative or integrative cancer clinics do offer many approaches and perhaps one would be perfect for you. Perhaps a raw vegan diet would work well for you; or perhaps you need a special diet that removes the triggers of your newly-discovered food allergies. Maybe vitamin B17 (also called Amygdalin) would melt your cancer away. Maybe some good Energy Medicine would hit the spot. We're all different and need a customized combination of treatments. So our first order of business is to get better acquainted with our bodies. That requires some time studying test results and understanding them with wise help from whomever we can find.

3. **Detoxifying**

We live in a toxic world these days. Whether we know it or not, our bodies are accumulating poisons from many sources:

- Polluted air – traffic fumes, factory smoke, agricultural spray poisons;

- Contaminated tap water – chlorine (a carcinogen) and fluoride (an endocrine disrupter); in some areas, drugs (legal and illegal) that got into the ground water and are not recognized by water companies;

- Processed and junk foods full of unresearched additives and known toxins;

- Fruits, vegetables and grain crops heavily sprayed with pesticides;

- GM crops (genetically modified), severely under-researched and potentially very destructive to health in lots of ways, especially for mothers and babies;

- High vibration radiation (e.g. cell phones and their towers, WIFI, and microwave ovens);

- Harmful chemicals in our household items (e.g. formaldehyde, a carcinogen, in carpets, curtains, clothing, plywood, adhesives, varnishes and wallpaper – it vaporizes at room temperatures and we breathe it in; and Perc (perchloroethylene), a carcinogenic solvent used in dry-cleaning that can leach into our skin or be breathed into our lungs, entering the bloodstream from both places.

Good health cannot be restored if these poisons are left in the body and allowed to continue accumulating. There are many simple and inexpensive ways to detoxify ourselves.

This Saga is about how I started in ignorance, taking my cancer symptom management pills every day, but grew into a persistent searcher for my own cancer cure. Along the way, I did my energy work as I had learned to do it in a California Institute I attended for about eight years and some chapters offer pieces of that energy information for those interested.

Note: The objective text interspersed with the book's narrative is marked before and after by this:

I hope this book helps you to avoid some of my mistakes and to successfully regain your good health. Please use the Memorandum after each chapter to note your own thoughts.

Here's a start:

Memorandum

✓

✓

✓

✓

Chapter 1: Diagnosis

The anesthesiologist hurried in and as she leaned to place the anesthetic mask over my face, she glanced at the paperwork in her other hand.

"Oh! No! No, we can't do this!"

The nurse was startled, as was I, but the anesthesiologist didn't explain.

"You need to see a doctor immediately, Ms. Kimberley. We'll make an appointment for you tomorrow."

They gave me the name of a doctor and his whereabouts and the appointment time.

I had moved to Colorado one year previously from California, the South Bay area. My husband of 11 years, Fred, had died of cancer just three months after his diagnosis. I was still mourning; but stumbling around in Denver, I got a job, got laid off, and was now unemployed. I had COBRA coverage, three months of government help with healthcare costs, and I'd decided to take this opportunity to have my deviated septum corrected. It would be easier to breathe at night if the two nostrils were equal in width. That plan was now defunct.

I shuffled to the appointment next day like some manniquin moved by remote control. I knew what the anesthesiologist had probably seen but wasn't verbalizing it to myself. The doctor, I'll call him Dr. Marconi, seemed to be a kindly man though he seemed in a perpetual hurry. He ordered a bone marrow biopsy for me to make sure that what I had was Chronic Myeloid Leukemia (CML). The Complete Blood Count (CBC) that had startled the anesthesiologist had shown a white cell count of 169,000 (per cc of blood). The normal range is 4,000 to 11,000.

This biopsy was done in Dr. Marconi's office a day or two later by his nurse practitioner. It's a procedure where a long hollow needle is pushed through a certain place on the hip bone into the marrow and a tiny piece of marrow is aspirated for testing. It was done with no anesthetic. The nurse was kind and meant well, but she had trouble getting the needle in correctly. So she had to try five times before the aspiration of marrow was successful.

By that time, I was so shaky and weak from pain that I couldn't sit up. They pulled me up and two nurses propped me up while another brought me a glass of water. When I could slide off the operating table, I got dressed and limped home for the several-week wait. Sure enough, the results showed the presence of Ph chromosomes – Philadelphia chromosomes, the defining mark of CML.

"I'm prescribing Gleevec for you, Jen," said Dr. Marconi on my follow-up appointment. It's made by Novartis, a Swiss company. Take one each day."

"How much does Gleevec cost? I lost my job."

"I have no idea. Talk to my nurse and she'll get you all the information you need. Or the social worker."

"How long might it take for Gleevec to cure the leukemia?"

"Since CML is chronic rather than acute, we can keep it under good control with Gleevec. It does have an acute phase at some point. The longest anyone with CML has lived from diagnosis is nine-and-a-half years. Get a CBC monthly and make an appointment to see me every three months." He raised his voice. "Next!"

No, he didn't actually call Next but his manner indicated that my time was up.

Nine-and-a-half years seemed a long time and since freedom from any health problems up to this point had convinced me that I'd live for at least 100 years like Auntie Dede, my first piano teacher, who lived to 101, I didn't worry. Yet. Talking to the social worker, I learned that a month's supply of Gleevec would cost about $8,500. No way! However, Novartis had a Patient Assistance program and being unemployed, I would qualify for it. She had me fill out a form and submit my previous year's tax return, and that was it. I think they gave me a bottle of Gleevec to cover me till the Novartis program got going and then bottles would arrive monthly in the mail.

Nobody offered to discuss why or how I might have gotten this leukemia, whether I'd had any exposure to radiation (I had) which is known to cause leukemia; and nobody checked my body's oxygen saturation or pH levels or asked about my diet. No tests were ordered to see if I had food allergies or any vitamin or mineral deficiencies. No ultrasound procedure was done to check on the normality of my abdominal organs. At the time, I'd never heard of links between any of those things and cancer. So in my ignorance I didn't feel neglected or short-changed; it just seemed that I'd struck a rocky patch on Life's path but soon I'd climb past it.

I'd had a series of radiation treatments 18 months previously. Before Fred was diagnosed with cancer, my ophthalmologist had diagnosed a cavernous sinus meningioma – a benign growth next to the left optic nerve. Treatment was planned but I put it aside when Fred was diagnosed. After he died I spent about nine months tying up loose ends and planning the move to Denver. One loose end was radiation treatments. They used four beams converging and five towards the end of the series. One went through the pituitary gland and another through the thyroid. They suggested I might have thyroid problems at some point but instead I think I got leukemia. (Narrative continues on p. 8)

What's in Blood?

A great deal is known about blood so this is a brief summary. We have on average about five liters (eleven pints) of blood continuously flowing through the body. Whole blood consists of a fluid called plasma with three kinds of cells (also called corpuscles) swimming in it. In a process called hematopoiesis, they are made from stem cells in the bone marrow where, normally, they grow to maturity and are then released into the bloodstream.

1. **Red cells** (erythrocytes) that carry hemoglobin on their membrane (outside surface), a protein that takes oxygen to all the body cells;

2. **Platelets** (thrombocytes) the smallest of the blood cells, necessary for clotting. If you sustain a break in the skin, they rush to the site and clump where a blood vessel has been broken. They act like the famous Dutch boy who put his finger in the dike but in reverse, stopping the flood from going out rather than from coming in. Thus they protect us from excessive bleeding.

3. **White cells** (leukocytes) that have several types and they all fight infection. The various types fall into two groups:

   ✓ **Granulocytes**, containing granules, which are enzymes on the outside skin (membrane) of the granulocyte that enable cell digestion of captured particles when the cell folds inwards over the captive:

➢ Neutrophils are the first to attack invading bacteria or fungi;

➢ Eosinophils focus mostly on parasites and allergens;

➢ Basophils focus largely on allergens but also some parasites, e.g. ticks.

✓ **Agranulocytes** (without granules)

➢ Lymphocytes work mainly in the lymph system; some are called Natural Killer cells (NK cells) as they need no antibodies helping them find the invaders. They're just "a natural" at the job. (See pp. 69-70 for more on lymphocytes.)

➢ Monocytes engulf and destroy pathogens;

➢ Macrophages also engulf and destroy pathogens and dead cell debris. They can pass through capillary walls, entering nearby tissue in pursuit of pathogens.

"Phagocytes" is another term for some white cells (neutrophils, eosinophils and monocytes) and there's a verb – they "phagocytose" microbes and dead particles. Leukemia is cancer of the white cells.

Blood Plasma

A bit over half the blood volume is plasma, the yellowish fluid that bathes and floats all the above cells. It's mostly water with some proteins. It carries all the dissolved components of our food:

o Glucose from carbohydrates;

o Amino acids from proteins; and

o Fatty acids from lipids.

It also carries waste products from cells (such as lactic acid, carbon dioxide and urea) and hormones taking messages to tissues around the body.

Blood Serum is plasma without the proteins involved with platelets in clotting. "Serum" is from the Latin word for "whey", as in "curds and whey". If you have ever made cheese, you know this because cheeses are made from curds.

Blood pH Value

Blood stays within a narrow range of pH (acidity/alkalinity). Seven is the neutral point, neither acid nor base (alkaline); blood is slightly basic, between 7.35 and 7.45. Saliva and urine pH can be measured at home with litmus paper and can vary around 7, but the body will always keep the blood at 7.35 to 7.45.

Hemoglobin

Blood gets its red color from the red cells, which in turn get their color from hemoglobin, a red molecule that carries oxygen. Arterial blood is bright red but venous blood is a dull red because waste products distort the color.

Blood Circulation

Arteries carry oxygen-loaded blood away from the heart and veins bring the waste-loaded blood back to it. Upon receiving venous blood, the heart sends it to the lungs via the pulmonary artery for clean-up. As we breathe oxygen (O_2) in and carbon dioxide (CO_2) out, the lungs are funneling venous blood through smaller and smaller vessels until it comes to tiny bronchioles, air sacs where CO_2 is exchanged for O_2.

Now, full of O_2, it's fresh arterial blood and works its way out of the lungs via larger and larger vessels until the pulmonary vein delivers it back to the heart. (This is the only instance of a vein carrying oxygen-loaded blood; all other veins carry waste-loaded venous blood.) The heart pumps the arterial blood into the large aorta, the artery that begins its new journey around the body. There are four chambers inside the heart, separated by a wall down the center and a valve dividing each side vertically. This accommodates all the blood's coming and going. Blood completes a full body run in three minutes or so.

Blood and the Liver

Along the way, it courses through the liver, depositing a) waste products for excretion through the colon and b) unfamiliar toxins for storage, not knowing what else to do with them. The liver also doesn't know what to do with them other than tuck them away in some corner. Over years and decades, if no detoxification is done, these old toxins build up, the liver forever dealing with more of them if nothing is done to improve the diet or toxic lifestyle. Eventually this overworked liver breaks down and the person has liver failure that soon causes death.

One good way to help both the blood and the liver with this toxin problem is coffee enemas. For more on this, see pp. 64-65.

Bone Marrow

Bone marrow is a spongy substance filling the cavities inside larger bones and it contains stem cells. Babies have active bone marrow in all their bones but adults have it only in the spinal bones, hips, shoulders, ribs, and skull. (Stem cell research is controversial but only concerning embryonic stem cells, which require an embryo to be killed, that is, an abortion.) Adult stem cells are not controversial and much research has been done on them worldwide. For more on stem cells, see Chapter 6.

Blood Cell Creation

Blood cells are created in bone marrow by stem cells. There are two kinds of those stem cells:

- o Lymphoid stem cells, which make the white cells called lymphocytes; and
- o Myeloid stem cells, which make red cells, platelets and the white cells called granulocytes and monocytes.

When new cells develop, they're at first immature, not looking like the cell type they're going to be and not yet able to do their job. These immature cells are called blast cells. Normally, blast cells remain in the bone marrow until they become mature. Then they're released into the blood to do their jobs. In Chronic Myeloid Leukemia, blast cells get into the blood and being counted as white cells they drive up the total white cell count.

Leukemia

Leukemia is cancer of the white blood cells (leukocytes) and since it features elevated white cell counts, the 19th century physicians who first observed it called it White Blood. Later, someone coined the term *leukemia* from Greek words meaning *white* and *blood*. (*cf. anemia*, low (absent) red cells)

Four Main Types of Leukemia

1. Chronic Myeloid (or Myelogenous) Leukemia (CML): slowly progressing and generated by myeloid stem cells

2. Acute Myeloid Leukemia (AML): Fast progressing;

3. Chronic Lymphocytic Leukemia (CLL). Slowly progressing and generated by lymphoid stem cells. Not to be confused with Lymphoma, which is cancer of the lymph system.

4. Acute Lymphocytic Leukemia (ALL): Fast progressing.

About Other Leukemias

All the leukemias feature elevated leukemic stem cell numbers that crowd the bone marrow and elevated white blood cell numbers that crowd the blood. This interferes with the functions of marrow and blood.

Leukemias are the most frequently-diagnosed of all cancers in children but 90% of leukemias occur in adults, not in children. The most common types in adults are AML and CLL.

All of the main four types of leukemia have sub-types. For CML, the sub-type is Chronic Monocytic Leukemia, cancer of the monocytes.

Leukemias and Other Cancers in Pets

Dogs, cats, and horses can all come down with cancer. Feline leukemia is caused by a virus that weakens the immune system, leaving the cat open to many other infections. Our pets live in the same environments we live in so surely the same toxins and radiation that contribute to human cancer also contribute to animal cancer. And surely the commercial animal foods we give to our pets also contribute, containing the same sorts of chemical additives as processed human food: artificial flavors and colors, hormones, preservatives, bulking agents, cheap chemical substitutes for Nature's ingredients, and so on.

We can probably protect our pets from cancer in the same ways we protect ourselves, especially pets that live in our house with us. Animals are closer to many poisons, e.g.

formaldehyde in carpets and drips or leaks from bottles of toxic household or yard cleaners. And as they're smaller, it takes smaller amounts of poison to sicken them.

Health food stores sell clean organic brands of pet food. There's also the option of making their meals from the same hormone-free, antibiotic-free, cage-free etc. ingredients that we use for ourselves. If we're vegetarian, we could add meats and fish from the local health food store.

Getting on With Life

Rather than focusing on my cancer diagnosis, I worked on building a new life in Denver. Since I had no tumors or pain, I didn't feel cancerous.

I had known nobody in Denver when I'd arrived but now a year later, I did have one new friend, Sue, my "dancing sister" (photo on p. 140). She had approached me at a dance studio where we were both having private lessons and together we must have gone to every dancing spot in greater Denver that offered West Coast Swing, Latin, Country, and Ballroom. I'd been a dance enthusiast since I was 20 and first moved to America. Living in Berkeley in 1963-66, I went every Friday night to the International Folk Dancing on campus. At the time, this was very popular and over the years I joined similar groups in Cambridge, MA and Sydney, Australia including a performing troupe, dancing at street fairs and ethnic clubs in Sydney. I love that Eastern European music with its odd rhythms – 5/8, 7/8 and 9/8.

Shortly after my diagnosis, I auditioned for the Colorado Symphony Chorus and sang with them for the next five years, working as a contract technical writer and editor.

One of my monthly blood tests displeased Dr. Marconi. I had not bothered to study or understand those tests. Looking back, I'm appalled at how cavalier I was about having cancer. It was the mix of at first grieving for Fred and not caring whether I lived or died; along with having no tumors or pain; and with enjoying my copious dancing and singing. The Chorus singing made up for not playing my fiddle. Since I was ten, I'd played violin, joining several local orchestras and also fiddling in small groups in street fairs and Irish pubs. But arthritis in my fingers made it impossible to play.

Apparently my white cell count had risen unacceptably, as shown in the CBC (Complete Blood Count), and Dr. Marconi decided that I'd become immune to Gleevec. A new alternative had come on the market shortly before called Sprycel, made by Bristol-Myers-Squibb, so he prescribed one of those daily. Being still unaware of the trouble this leukemia would cause, I took Sprycel as ordered and continued my new life for three more years. I was proud and pleased with myself for building it from scratch because my social skills had been non-existent until I cobbled something together in my 30s and 40s. It's harder to learn something years after the developmental stage for it has passed. My growing-up years were not conducive to making or retaining friends.

Hulda Clark

Specifically what started me on exploring alternative cancer care, I can't recall. But something started me googling around and in 2009 I came upon my first guru in curing cancer: Dr. Hulda Clark.

I read her book, *The Cure For All Cancers* and implemented many of the lifestyle changes she recommends. Her over-arching theory is that all diseases arise from the combination of toxins in our environment and parasites in our body. When I applied that to my own cancer, I realized that I was continually contributing to it by using toxic house-cleaning products, possibly toxic personal care products, and tap water which probably contained chlorine, an established carcinogen. I recalled with dismay the many times I'd swum in chlorinated swimming pools or soaked in chlorinated hot tubs, not to mention taken countless showers under chlorinated tap water. I resolved to eliminate all the chief suspects from my life and thus hopefully motivate the troops supposed to be protecting me from leukemia. So I started following her recommendations on how to replace the toxic items:

- I kept a supply of grain alcohol (same as vodka but cheaper) diluted, and used it 50% as a spray to clean room air; for cleaning sinks, sink drains, and

> To keep the body in good health is a duty... otherwise we shall not be able to keep our mind strong and clear.
>
> ---Buddha

counters; also in a shallow little bowl at food prep time to clean beneath my fingernails; also in a bowl of water to clean vegetables.

- I stopped buying all the other cleaners with their less-than-healthy chemicals and possibly heavy metals.

- I stopped using the microwave oven as it kills nutrients.

Eliminating poisons from the home is an essential step in any cancer recovery. Another essential step is eliminating poisons from the body. I started this with Hulda Clark's liver cleanse. Twice, I assembled all the ingredients, printed out the instructions, and followed them to the letter. What dramatic results! Hundreds of greenish or tan lumps floating in the bowl along with assorted sticks, flaps, and other unidentifiable debris and a number of what looked like worms between about one inch long and four or five inches long. (For more on worms, see p. 177)

Hulda Clark explained how the liver works hard continuously to clear our bodies of toxins. If we continually ingest contaminated foods and drinks such as supermarkets sell, and never do any detoxification, the liver can eventually become too overloaded to do its job effectively and too full of stored toxins to accommodate any more. That causes toxins to build up in the body fat and other tissues, creating a wide assortment of ill health conditions. The plethora of toxins can also overwhelm the immune system and cause it to shut down.

I also made a Zapper and used it daily to kill off any parasites in my body. This was an early form of what is now called Energy Medicine, where various types of machines emit vibrations that match the targeted pathogen, thus killing it. That was also how Dr. Royal Rife killed the pleomorphic microbes that his powerful and well-designed microscope enabled him to see live inside cancer cells. He ascertained their specific vibrational speed and matched it with his Rife Machine. (For more on Royal Rife, see pp. 11-13)

My time in Colorado was coming to an end. I was aware now that my immune system was somehow damaged, but what exactly the immune system consisted of, beyond "white cells", I didn't yet know. I've never been one to get a lot of colds; have never had the flu; and other than an obstetrician for each baby, never had a doctor before my cancer doctor. So I didn't feel threatened or at risk because my immunity was compromised – I just had the concept of being deficient in functioning white cells.

In fact, before I had lost my second husband, Fred, to lung cancer, I had lost my younger brother in Australia to stomach cancer and my mother to oral cancer. Still, I didn't feel threatened by cancer myself. If it had been a tumorous cancer, perhaps it would have been more frightening and could have caused me a lot of pain. I was fortunate that my leukemia caused no pain at all but now it was starting to cause fatigue.

I had to withdraw from the Colorado Symphony Chorus. Whenever we had concerts, there would be an extra rehearsal that week as well as two or three concerts that weekend and that was too much for me. I couldn't help but get dazed with fatigue half-way through each evening. I was holding down a full-time job by then as the lead in-house writer at a website development company. It was a hard and sad decision but it was necessary and spurred me on to find a cure for this pesky cancer. (Narrative continues on p. 13)

Dr. Royal Raymond Rife, 1888 to 1971

Dr. Royal Rife was raised by an aunt after his mother died when he was a baby. He was known as Roy Rife among his friends and colleagues. In 1905 when he was 17, he wanted to be a doctor and enrolled at Johns Hopkins University but before long, his interest had shifted to bacteriology and then also optics. After studying at Johns Hopkins, he invented a series of devices, many of which are still used – technology in optics, aviation, radiochemistry, electronics, and biochemistry. For all this accomplishment he was given 14 major awards, and from the University of Heidelberg (where he worked for a few years), an honorary doctorate in 1914.

Watching Live Viruses in his Universal Microscope

In 1912, aged 24, he married a young woman named Mamie Quinn who was his loyal and supportive wife until her death in 1957. They had no children. By the age of 32, he had created the first microscope powerful enough to reveal viruses and he became the first person ever to see one. By the age of 45, he had perfected it as the Rife Universal Microscope and it could magnify objects by 60,000 times their original size. Not only could it show viruses, but they were live viruses – other microscopes could see only dead things, since the things to be examined are stained first, which kills live creatures. (A dark field microscope can see live things – e.g., see p. 141) All microscopes need a light to make things visible. Dr. Rife's microscope used ultraviolet light, a range of frequencies that are too short to be visible. But he used two different wavelengths of ultraviolet light, that, when colliding with each other, created a third, longer frequency that is visible. Now the microbes were visible and still alive.

Dr. Rife could see viruses moving around and he studied their movements, recording their different frequencies of vibration. He agreed with those who propounded Pleomorphism – the ability of microbes to change their shape and structure multiple times, responding to changes in their immediate microscopic environment.

Killing Viruses in Diseased Tissue

All molecules on planet Earth vibrate at certain frequencies. This fact underlies Hulda Clark's Synchrometer, used to detect specific chemicals in such things as hand lotion or laundry detergent. It also underlies the famous scenario of a soprano singer breaking a wine glass -- her pitch vibration coincides with the glass molecule vibration and by adding to it, causes an excess of vibration that shatters the glass.

Although Dr. Rife's microbes were alive under his microscope, he also developed a technique to kill them in diseased tissue. He could see the herpes virus, polio virus, those of influenza and tetanus, and among others, those of cancer. He worked for years pinpointing all these vibrational frequencies, then applied the same frequencies in his microscope to destroy the microbes.

To treat live humans, he developed the Rife Frequency Machine and a magazine article about it was published in 1931. It operated on the same principle of matching vibrations and is seen now as a forerunner of today's Energy Medicine. By applying specific electro-magnetic vibrations, this machine could kill microbes without affecting the surrounding healthy tissue. During his development of this machine, Rife used it on 16 cancer patients, curing all of them 100%. These 16 cures were documented at the time by a team of doctors who had initially diagnosed these patients as being "terminal".

In 1934, a group of doctors and bacteriologists treating terminally ill cancer patients worked with Dr. Rife in San Diego for three months. The Rife Machine was used to kill cancer microbes painlessly and the cancer was found to then be reversible. After one or in some cases two treatments, all patients were cancer-free.

This caused a nationwide storm with newspapers, medical journals and conferences. In 1939 Dr. Rife's career was ended though he lived to 1971. This Saga cannot tell you the rest of the sad and outrageous story but it is related in detail in *The Cancer Cure That Worked* by Barry Lynes, listed in this Saga's Print and PDF Resources.

Devices called Rife Machines have lately become available. They vary in how they operate and perform and may or may not resemble Dr. Rife's original machines. Nobody has managed to reconstruct his microscope as there are no documents left for guidance; they were all destroyed but not by Dr. Rife.

Energy Work #1: Grounding

Back in May 1978, I walked into an Institute in Berkeley and thus ended a big Search that had started when I was 13. I'd been looking for someone to teach me how to meditate. I'd tried various religious groups and several books, but all to little effect. Now in this Institute I found dozens of people who could teach me. I signed up for the Meditation I class.

Since grounding is so basic to effective energy work, the next few pages present my memory of that first class that totally turned me around. I would be long dead now if it hadn't been for what I was taught at that Institute. Though this book is about cancer, it's also about how I dealt with my cancer. Grounding and energy work have been central and effective in enabling me to cope and stay strong. I believe they can be effective for anyone at any time, especially a cancer patient trying to sort through the jumble of emotions, advice, and possible choices.

As I waited the three weeks for class to start, I went to healing clinics and spent time at the Institute sipping coffee and listening to people talk. I learned that the area around my body is not empty – it's my aura, my spirit energy. We human beings are not just bodies; we are spirits living in bodies. We live in them for a time and then we leave and go Home. Back to where we came from. I knew this already as I'd had many experiences as a child that floated me to the spirit world at bedtime and healed me of each day's wounds.*

Auras can be healed – they can be photographed too, as I learned a little later at a Psychic Fair in the Berkeley Veterans' Hall. Someone had a kirlean camera and my aura showed up as very green with areas of orange and yellow and bits of blue, each color merging gently into the others.

When Meditation I started, with about 30 students, the first thing we learned was how to ground ourselves.

"Put your feet flat on the floor," said Kathy, our young teacher, (not her real name), wife of one of the other staff members. She was slim and had shiny round eyes, round cheeks and a happy smile.

We were in the living room of an old house. Bright light from the front bow windows filled the room and the closed side door to the front entryway still allowed us to hear the muted voices of people chatting and laughing on the front porch.

"Get comfortable in your chair," – we had folding metal chairs though some sat on the two couches – "and rest your hands in your lap, palms up."

There was a bit of shuffling and throat-clearing as people settled in. Looking around, I noticed how young everyone was. It was early June 1978 and I was about to turn 36. The others looked to be in their twenties or teens and seemed unburdened, as if a Spring breeze could puff them away. I felt heavy with divorce grief and motherhood worries.

"Now close your eyes and relax." Kathy paused.

"We have seven major chakras energy centers, in the body. The first chakra is at the base of the spine. Feel your tail bone, your "sitz bones", where your chair supports you.

"Imagine a line running from this first chakra clear to the center of planet Earth. Don't try hard. Postulate this line. Imagine it as a sturdy tree trunk or big tap root or an elevator shaft. Whatever image comes to you.

"This line is an energy cord – a Grounding Cord. You can give it a color, or not. Just let it drop down to the center of the planet."

---

* For more about this, please see *Poems For Your Heart*, Jen Kimberley, Balboa Press, 2017

Kathy walked slowly around the room as she talked, observing each of us.

"You can anchor it by tucking it beneath a big rock or a pile of small rocks or just postulate that it is self-anchored. Just form the notion that it reliably and comfortably connects your first chakra to the center of the earth.

"Sit for a few minutes enjoying its presence. Be pleased with yourself for having it. The more often you do this, the easier it becomes to create and the more effective it becomes in grounding you."

I had mine like a waterfall and I tucked it under a boulder.

"Grounding cords are not just nice assets or decorations. They're to be used. They enable you to release unwanted energy any time. If you feel bothered by some situation or condition in your life, postulate that it's going down your grounding cord Let go of it. Many of us find it hard to let go of things – we're energy pack rats and some of us lug around increasing loads of other people's energy our entire lives. But letting go is a terrific feeling, an increased feeling of freedom, of lightness, of your sense of self. So any preoccupation or worry that's on your mind can be released down the grounding cord."

A voice spoke up. "I want my mother's energy to go down the grounding cord. Will that make her worry and call me up to fuss?"

Kathy laughed, as did some others. "No. If it involves someone else, it won't hurt them. It's not disloyal or uncooperative. It's just being more yourself. The other person is equally free to let go of your energy if they've been carrying some of it around.

"When we let go of unwanted energy in this way and it falls to the center of the planet, it becomes neutralized. Once you let it go, it's no longer "your" energy, cluttering up your space. It gets recycled. It becomes nobody's own energy, just universally available energy. Without it, you now have more freedom to run your own energy through your body. Keeping your body grounded is protective. It takes away jumpiness and anxiety and promotes calm."

Years later, when I lived in Denver, I had a young co-worker, (I'll call him Harry), with a big playful streak who liked to creep up behind you and suddenly say something loud. He enjoyed triggering the startle response. Most people took it with good grace. They jumped or gave a little shriek and turned around and then laughed and patted their chest. In my case, it didn't work. A grounded body doesn't startle. You hear the sudden sound but that sound energy flows uneventfully down your grounding cord and your body is unaffected. Harry was baffled. He kept trying for weeks and I said,

"I've got grounding, Harry. I keep myself grounded." I thought he might get the idea from thinking of grounding wires in a house. But it didn't mean anything to him. Eventually he gave up but we still got along fine.

Sometimes I'm not as well-grounded as I like to be and something does startle me. Then I let go of whatever grounding I do have, let it disconnect from the first chakra and fall away; then I create a new grounding cord. It's good to refresh your grounding often and keep it in present time.

Replenish With a Gold Sun

Letting energy leave your space creates gaps and it's important to fill them. They'll get filled by someone else if not by you and you don't want to invite others to put their energy in your space. A gold sun is the other side of the grounding coin. Imagine your gold sun above your head, bright and fresh and filled with your own creative energy. Let it shine down into all your chakras, your whole body, even your grounding cord. Take your time and feel the gratifying sensation of your own energy fueling your whole being. Own that energy. It's yours and it's there for you to create a life with.

Each color is an energy level, a vibrational level, and gold is a high vibration. It's not a coincidence that royalty everywhere covets and displays gold on their person and in their surroundings. Some people use white energy to fill up with and that's good too; white is a high energy and contains all colors. It's associated with purity, as in clergy vestments and traditional wedding gowns. I like to use gold because it's a warm color and good for filling the fourth chakra, the heart chakra.

This world so much needs love but where do we get it from? Do we go "Looking for love in all the wrong places", as the old song went? *

No, we:

> "Seek and [we] shall find,
> Ask and it shall be given,
> Knock and the door shall be opened
> And the love comes a trickling down." **

We welcome it into our own heart as gold energy. Then we can share it. Don't we love people who have "a heart of gold"? And as another song says:

> "Some say love it is a hunger,
> An endless aching need;
> I say love, it is a flower,
> **And you its only seed**." ***

Grounding Through the Feet

You don't need to buy any electrical or magnetic devices when grounding from the first chakra. That grounding becomes part of your energy being; it travels with you and is always working for you as long as you refresh it regularly and keep it in present time. It drains off pain and tension and improves your sleep.

By bringing you more into your body and keeping you more relaxed, it can improve every aspect of health.

There is also the barefoot method called earthing. You can ground both ways simultaneously. Walk barefoot on the grass or soil or sand. It's great to feel that earth energy enter your feet chakras and flow up the leg channels. Most children know all

---

* Written by Wanda Mallette, Bob Morrison and Patti Ryan; recorded by Johnny Lee; released June 1980 as part of the soundtrack of the movie Urban Cowboy. https://www.youtube.com/watch?v=I2689Izx2UQ

** Traditional gospel song arranged and sung by various people, e.g. Shawn Phillips on his album "Shawn", released in 1965. https://www.youtube.com/watch?v=vOO_r-A_xVE

*** The Rose, copyright © 1978, Bette Midler; music and lyrics by Amanda McBroom https://www.youtube.com/watch?v=zxSTzSEiZ2c

about it through their as-yet-uncrushed right brain instinct. It brings you more into the body, your home for the current lifetime.

We the spirits living in these bodies don't belong to Earth but our bodies do and they feel gratified and validated when that connection is strengthened, whichever method you use. Surely one of the pleasures of this life is a barefoot run along the sand or over the grass, especially if your doggie runs with you.

Camouflage

Do moods and motives create our face?
Does the person we've been for all these years
Chisel and chip, twist and snip,
Paint our aging portrait?

No doubt; but there's more to the story.
Surely we have two kindly foes,
Two treacherous friends
Who help.

A cheering sun who greens the earth,
Coaxes crocuses,
Draws up daffodils,
Whispers encouragement to unfulfilled seeds;
His sub-plot slowly shows itself
As he toasts our willing faces
Till they match the wind-blown sand
And the dried-up Autumn weeds.

And our earth, that feeds and sings to us,
Grounding us to reality,
Who croons with the voice of honey bees,
Of mountain streams, of rustling trees,
Of crickets and birds and the cool night breeze –

She loves us and she wants us near,
Closer with every passing year.
We can't refuse; our bodies are hers
And little by piece they obey.

Our true self is hidden by our sun's handiwork,
Masked by our earth's possessive love;
But it's there for those
Who look to see
The spirit smiling through.

   ---Jen Kimberley, *Poems For Your Heart*, Balboa Press, 2017, p. 44

Memorandum

- ✓ We all have cancer cells; keep your immune system healthy so it can chase them down and dispose of them.
- ✓ Question your doctor. Get second, even third opinions and take time to digest new information.
- ✓ Search around on any topics that puzzle you and see if there's controversy, and if so, study each side to see which is most applicable to you.
- ✓ Read any literature your doctor gives you and mark places that raise questions. Get your questions clear and ask them on your next visit. If your doctor lacks time or inclination to answer them, find another doctor.
- ✓ To facilitate recovery from serious disease like cancer, one should detoxify the body and the home. We have control over those two areas whereas we can't necessarily avoid breathing in traffic fumes, for example.
- ✓ Stay grounded and filled up with your own gold creative energy. It will help you stay confident of recovering.
- ✓
- ✓
- ✓

Chapter 2: A Wake-up Call

By 2010 I felt my life priorities starting to change. Arthritis blocked violin playing, leukemia pushed me out of the Symphony chorus, my doctor rejected any cancer approaches other than the drug. I did still dance every weekend and work my job – I was the lead in-house writer at a website development company. And I had a nice house that I shared with my two cats and a young couple who rented the apartment above the free-standing garage. But each day, cancer loomed larger, demanding to become a higher priority.

In my previous travels I had spent some time in the Doninican Republic. It was a loose community with people coming and going and I had formed a friendship with Greg, a Canadian and a very capable carpenter. He had been reviving a carpentry area in an abandoned garage. He'd bought new tools and made a wall of hooks and shapes to store them on. Then he'd proceeded to make badly-needed cupboards, shelves and towel rails for the compound. He attracted several young local men who became his apprentices. Greg didn't speak Spanish but he was a genius at communicating without it and down in that garage there was a lot of laughing and learning.

Now, feeling that it was time to leave Denver and find some alternative cancer care, I emailed Greg and we arranged for me to visit him in Canada. He had experience with cancer as his grandson had been diagnosed with bone cancer at the age of seven. He'd done a lot of reading to find alternative ways to treat the child so I knew he was rather familiar with treatment choices for cancer. He picked me up at the airport and we drove to his house "at the lake", outside Moose Jaw, Saskatchewan. I always grinned inwardly at a town being called Moose Jaw. But it's not as if no other places have amusing names – there's my beloved childhood summer resort called Woy Woy and the surf beach in Sydney called Curl Curl, and the inland town called Wagga Wagga (pronounced Wogga Wogga) on the Murrumbidgee river. And there are the amazing Bungle Bungles in NW Australia … Well, I'm a wordsmith and love them all. I had a high school friend from a town called Come-by-Chance that had five houses, one shop and one petrol station … OK, back to Canada.

Greg and I drove into Moose Jaw many days and met up with his friends and I found a doctor and had a blood test done, a Complete Blood Count (CBC). It showed the white cells at 54 (54,000 white cells per cc of blood). The normal range is 4,000 to 11,000.

"Do you think my white count is too high, Doctor?"

"Oh no. It's nothing to worry about. Just keep doing what you're doing and get another test in a month or so."

When I'd been taking Gleevec and Sprycel for those eight years in Denver, I'd had monthly blood tests and had taken little notice of the results. In the quarterly doctor visits, my liver and spleen were palpated to see if they were getting enlarged (by stored, dead cancer cells – they never were), and the doctor glanced at the blood test results. Apparently they were always OK, as I don't recall him ever commenting. So because of my past lack of interest in blood test results, I had little idea of how high the white count could go and still be "nothing to worry about". So I didn't worry, and in my ignorance about any need for an anti-cancer diet, I continued eating as I had for years:

- Coffee with flavored coffee creamer,

- Fried eggs and hash browns with cheese and bacon;

- Fried meat and vegetable concoctions (that's my cooking style – I don't much follow recipes);

- Occasional salads, fruit and fish;

- Occasional alcoholic drinks.

Frying is not necessarily harmful but I ruined it by using the supermarket canola oil. More on canola oil in Chapter 5. The salads were not half often enough and the dressings were commercial, loaded with sugar, preservatives and other chemicals like fake flavors and colors. And nothing was organic.

In the ten Denver years, I had bought sweet treats like a cream puff, chocolate éclair, cheesecake or tiramisu, from the Whole Foods bakery, enjoying them with a cappuccino (sugared). That bakery dazzled me, so rich and colorful it was that I couldn't look without succumbing to something. I went there for my weekly fresh-baked loaf of sourdough French bread and stayed for the sweet treat.

On annual visits to my Dad in Sydney, I wandered around downtown, astounded at all the changes since I had been a university student there. I felt how much change had happened inside me too, such that I could now hug myself, so to speak, and smilingly love everything I looked at; whereas 40 years previously I could only plod and weep, at a loss for how to improve life. I had now vastly improved my life in many ways but not vis-à-vis diet. In Sydney, I continued the Denver sugar foolishness, sitting at an outdoor café table sipping sweetened cappuccinos and munching sweet treats, with a good book ready if I wanted it. I'd better not mention the frequent hot fudge sundaes with extra whipped cream that dated back to 1978.

However, I was never fond of canned, packaged, or frozen food and disliked all candy except dark chocolate. Growing up, I had been fed from our garden and fruit trees, eggs from our own chooks, all the cooking done by my mother with my help as I grew. I wasn't fat. No-one in my family has ever been fat. But I was certainly ignorant about how to eat when you have cancer. I hadn't yet caught on to the fact that an unhealthy diet and lifestyle are big contributing causes of cancer.

A Good Protocol Half-Done

The next CBC, three months later, showed the white count at about 100,000 – double the previous result. Again, the doctor said it was not enormously high and to just keep on with what I was doing.

However, I had continued reading online about alternative cancer treatments and had come upon Bill Henderson's protocol. Bill Henderson was not a doctor but became interested in alternative cancer care when he lost his wife to cancer. He worked as a coach with many hundreds of cancer patients and in return, over the years, received tons of happy Thank Yous. From his website, he offered individual counseling and became a prominent person in the world of alternative cancer care.

I started eating a blended mix of cottage cheese and flaxseed oil every day. This part of his protocol is borrowed from the Budwig diet. See pp. 24-5 and p. 85 for more on the Budwig Blend.

I also did daily vegetable juicing with many carrots in with the beetroot, celery, cabbage and cucumbers, etc. However, I didn't do juicing to anything like the extent advocated by the Gerson protocol which calls for 13 glasses of carrot juice daily, along with five coffee enemas. You need someone helping you with it. It involves other things too, and if they accept you, you can go with a friend or relative to their institute in Tijuana and learn all the details first-hand.

However, on the Bill Henderson protocol, I had one or two glasses of mostly-carrot juice daily. I also took a multi-vitamin-mineral tablet that he recommended and Beta-Glucan tablets daily. Beta-1, 3D Glucan binds to receptors on the outside of our neutrophils, activating them to recognize cancer cells as invaders to be destroyed. Otherwise, they don't see cancer cells as harmful though other white cells do. This doubles our immune system's effectiveness. (See pp. 3-6 for information on blood cells)

There is more to the Bill Henderson protocol but I didn't include it. Although I now had a big salad every day, I still used commercial dressings and had coffee with flavored creamer and a breakfast fried in canola oil. I enjoyed life, meeting Greg's friends and riding around on an ATV on the prairies. After three more months, I had a third CBC done and it showed my white count to be about 150,000. Still the doctor said not to worry. So I didn't and in December 2011, Greg and I took a plane to Costa Rica. At this point, I went off the Bill Henderson protocol, at least, off that part of it I'd been on. (Narrative continues on p. 25)

The Budwig Blend

First, some background facts.

o Cancer occurs when the body's oxygen supply is insufficient, a condition known as hypoxia. This was discovered by one Dr. Otto Warburg, a prominent German cell biologist studying cancer, and in 1931 he was given the Nobel Prize for it.

o Cancer can be reversed by raising the body's oxygen supply in a way that delivers the oxygen right into body cells.

o Natural plant oil molecules consist of an atom surrounded by a cloud of electrons that enable the molecules to be oxygenated, i.e., to bind with oxygen. Plants absorb and store the sun's energy, making it into food for animals (including us human animals).

o The plant oils most efficient in storing the sun's energy contain Omega 3 and Omega 6 fatty acids.

Johanna Budwig was a prominent German research chemist who lived 1906 to 2003. In the 1930s, 40s and 50s, everyone thought that an oil was just an oil. However, Dr. Budwig's years of analyzing oils, including all the processed oils in supermarkets, showed her that oils differ dramatically in their makeup and effects on our health. She discovered the Omega 3 and Omega 6 fatty acids that we now are so familiar with.

She also found that any diet using processed oils is lacking in linoleic acids. This absence causes the body to produce oxidase which supports cancer and many of our modern diseases.

Being a compatriot of Dr. Otto Warburg, she knew that body cells go cancerous when oxygen is lacking and her further research led her to think that if we could make natural plant oils, with their abundant oxygen and nutrition, water-soluble, they'd be able to enter body cells easily and by providing oxygen be able to revert cancer cells to normalcy.

She chose flaxseed oil to work with because of its high levels of Omega 3 and Omega 6 fatty acids and looked for a protein containing sulphur. That combination would make the oil water-soluble. She chose quark, the German version of cottage cheese. When she gave this blend of quark and flaxseed oil to cancer patients, their tumors shrank and their health greatly improved. She went on to devise an entire Budwig Diet which is still used successfully at various cancer clinics. Some cancer protocols use just the Budwig Blend, such as the Bill Henderson protocol.

Postscript #1: Dr. Budwig was nominated seven times for the Nobel Prize for her amazing work on oils and her success with cancer. But it was blocked each time.

Postscript #2: When fully blended with flaxseed oil, the cottage cheese loses its dairy properties, becoming harmless to people with a sensitivity to dairy products. I'm one such person and have had no problem with my months of Budwig Blend. For more on making the Budwig Blend, see p. 86.

My father had left me some money and I had used some of it to buy land. It was on the Caribbean side of Costa Rica. I wanted to create a homestead for my sons to visit or even live in. I planned to grow my own vegetables as my father had and his father before him; have some chooks for a supply of eggs; plant many fruit trees – avocado, mango, paw paw, lemon, banana, orange; perhaps eventually have two beehives. (The bees disappearing from Earth worries me.)

Greg had come with me partly to see Costa Rica and partly to design a floor plan for my house. He had good CAD-CAM skills. The first month we rented a room in Cahuita, on the second floor of a small hotel, with a balcony. It was a sleepy town. A busload of tourists arrived about once a week; they stayed overnight in a small hotel across from ours, then left the next morning. We got to know some local people and some long-term visitors from other countries. We also went to my land and though it was the wet season and very muddy, we put four stakes to mark where we thought the house would be best located.

After a month or so, we met a woman who owned a lodge at Puerto Viejo, further south on the coast from Cahuita and we moved into a room there for another month or so. It's a lovely town on the beach with one main street, lined with stalls selling bamboo furniture, straw hats, and hand-made clothing and jewelry, and interspersed among these are nice coffee shops and cafes. There are no large hotels as this part of Costa Rica caters to hitchhikers and backpackers who stay in small hostels and lodges.

Our lodge owner was singing in a small choir and invited me to join. She got around in a golf cart so we chugged along one night to a hostel lobby and there was a woman with a digital piano laid out on two chairs, facing five or six other women on a couch and easy chairs. She turned out to be the conductor and accompanist.

"We're practicing for an Easter concert," she said. "There are two other small groups and we'll come together at Easter. What part do you sing?"

"Alto."

Several women said, "Oh!" and "Ah", and one came over to sit next to me on the second couch.

"We've been needing more altos," she said. "We're starting with Mozart's Ave Verum Corpus."

I knew this ethereally beautiful short piece and my heart grew as big as an ocean as we sang through it. It's written for four parts so we were just rehearsing the two women's parts. As our conductor finished playing the accompaniment after the choral parts were finished, I watched her hands. She played beautifully, very subtle and strong. At the last chord, she looked up at me and our eyes locked. We each saw what a music lover the other was and I felt I had met a new friend. We went to these rehearsals several more times in the golf cart but I did not make it to the concert.

Turned 180 Degrees

Greg and I were going out for dinner each night in Cahuita and had a few favorite restaurants, simple local places.

"Greg," I said one night, "These chairs get harder every time we eat out. Have you noticed that?"

He looked bemused and said something vague. But I felt it acutely – discomfort on all the café chairs that seemed to slowly increase over these two months or so. I wasn't connecting the puzzle pieces, but soon life would connect them for me. After we'd been a month at the Puerta Viejo lodge, Greg decided to return to Canada and get a job. So we found a small cottage for me to rent and shortly after that, Greg left.

A day or two later, I was sitting on the side of my bed, laptop on my lap, writing emails, and I began to feel strange. Weak or vague. I disregarded it and finished the email and sent it. It was March 20, 2012.

Suddenly I was lying on the bed on my right side with my feet still on the floor. The Mac was half on my twisted lap but about to fall off. "What am I doing?" I thought. I sat up and retrieved it but as I looked around the room, my head spun. Alarmed, I put the Mac on the bedside table and lay fully on the bed on my left side, facing the door, head on the pillow. Each time I moved my head, the room bounced and rocked. But I felt no pain.

I lay wondering what had happened to me and eventually my landlady came by, I forget why. She had two young children and was 8 months pregnant. She and her family lived on the same acre or so of land, their house about 20 yards from my cottage. She spoke English well. I'll call her Mary and her husband Juan.

"I can't sit up, Mary," I said. "The world bounces when I move." She was a warm-hearted woman and immediately became concerned.

"Did you fall? Are you hurt?" she asked.

"Only fell on the bed. No, not hurt."

She fetched her husband Juan, a quiet man from Spain who was an architect and had built the beautiful cottage I was in.

"I'll have a doctor come and see you," he said.

Soon a local doctor did arrive with his traditional doctor's bag. He sat on my bed and asked questions in his excellent English, then gave me a brief examination with stethoscope, thermometer, etc. I showed him the bloodwork results that I'd had done after I arrived in Costa Rica, showing a very elevated white cell count. I believe it was about 600,000 per cc of blood, up from the 150,000 it had been when I left Canada three months previously.

"Jen, I think you had a mild stroke. It might have been from a virus or it might have been your leukemia. Something blocked some little capillaries in your brain."

I stared at him at a loss. Then I remembered my first cancer doctor telling me back in 2001 that Chronic Myeloid Leukemia (CML) has an acute phase after being chronic for years, and when it switches into its acute phase, conventional doctors cannot help. He also had said that the longest anyone with CML had lived after diagnosis was 9.5 years. It was now 10.5 years since my diagnosis (November 2001 to March 2012). "The leukemia's gone acute," I thought. So that was my reading of this situation and I saw that I'd better find someone who could help or this bed I was in would be my last.

Two days after I lost my balance, I also lost much of my hearing. The left ear (as was diagnosed later in Arizona) lost three quarters of its hearing and the right ear lost about one quarter. I began to feel despondent. As a lifetime musician and dancer, I could not have lost two more important functions than hearing and balance. Lying in that cottage bed, I realized that I'd need to reserve all my remaining inherited money for cancer treatments, wherever I would be able to get them. I had no health insurance, as I'd given it up when I left my job in Colorado. I would have to pay out of pocket.

No Go at Gerson

I called the Gerson Institute in Tijuana and at their request, had a copy of my recent blood work results mailed to them. They turned me down as being too sick. Well, that was upsetting but I thought at the time that it did make sense, as the Gerson method apparently takes two years or so and depends a lot on the 13 glasses of carrot juice and five coffee enemas daily along with selected supplements and specially-prepared food. People need a long-term helper like a parent, spouse or adult child. I had no helpers and needed something faster than that. Later, I learned that the Gerson clinic takes end-stage cancer patients all the time so that leaves me puzzled as to why they turned me down. But never mind; it's moot now.

A Solution in Arizona

Greg came to my rescue by suggesting that I try An Oasis of Healing, an alternative cancer clinic in Arizona. He knew about it from the research he'd done when his grandson had been diagnosed. From my bed in the cottage, I called them and spoke to a young, friendly woman whose job it was to interview people over the phone and accept or reject them. Oasis rejects virtually nobody except children as they're not equipped to treat them. So she accepted me over the phone and asked me to fax my blood work results, which Juan did for me. The founder and director of Oasis, Dr. Thomas Lodi, would look at the blood work and be ready for me when I arrived.

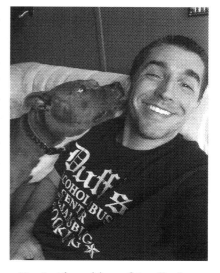

Dmitri loved by a friend's dog.

---Photo by Dmitri

Now the question was how to get there. My son, Dmitri, stepped up for this. He has a high pressure job in New York as a website programmer responsible for many deadlines. He was about to finish a six-year project he'd had, managing a team of programmers who created a website for a big client.

While he took care of the last bits of that job, Mary took care of me. She brought me three nutritious meals each day and sat with me to talk. Her company was enormously comforting. She was a gentle woman who understood the rather desperate situation I was in.

The cottage had a kitchen, bedroom and bathroom with the kitchen and bedroom opening separately from the common patio. To get to the bathroom, I had to crawl, taking a pillow with me. After each inch forward, I stopped to rest my head on the pillow until it slowed its bouncing enough for the next inch.

Departure From Costa Rica

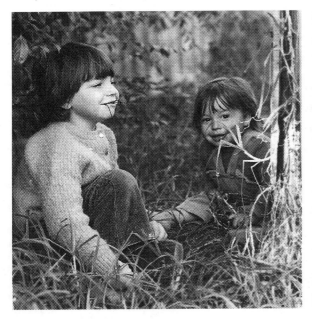

Chris and Dmitri in our yard, Sydney, 1975, ages 6 and 2

Photo by Jen Kimberley

Dmitri rented a car at the San Jose airport and drove down to the Caribbean coast. That's a white-knuckle drive as the road is just two lanes most of the way; it makes many hairpin curves above dramatic drop-offs into jungle ravines; it lacks lighting, signs, and side barriers; it has patches where the road has crumbled away at the edge; and it is jam-packed with big rigs. Rather than creep along behind a big rig, many drivers dart out and pass without being able to see the oncoming traffic. If you drive that way and survive, it's a five to six-hour trip. Dmitri chose not to take those risks, especially as daylight faded, so it took him a full day to get to my cottage.

Dmitri is my second son. He was born in Australia and came with me to California when he was four. He was an easy birth and a sunny-natured child. He adored his big brother Chris and when they left for school together each day, he looked out for him.

"Have you got your homework Chris?"

"Have you got your lunch money?"

As often as not, Chris didn't, and went back inside for the missing items. Chris was a happy child too and entertained Dmitri with his antics and improvised games. Now Dmitri lives in New York City, plays guitar and sings in a band, and works to a high standard at his programming job. He is also proficient in Photoshop, his favorite software and mine too.

When he arrived, he took over the food preparation. I could now stand up for a short while if I held on to something and didn't move, but turning and leaning over were out of the question. So Dmitri packed two suitcases for me and explained to my landlord and landlady that he was taking me to America for cancer treatment.

I paid them advance rent into August, expecting to be back by then and wanting to stay in the cottage. How little I knew. They offered to pack away the things I had to leave behind and keep them safe from mold and insects. When I had sold my house in Denver, I had let go of many possessions but had kept the most important like old photos and letters, the astrological chart that my grandmother did when I was born, music I'd written or arranged, books such as a beautiful big anatomy book and an atlas, and some appliances such as my ozonator, sewing machine, printer, and bread machine. And of course my guitar and flute. Now I had to leave all these valued things behind. Though I knew that cancer treatments paid for out of pocket would deplete the money my Dad had left me, I still hoped to return by August and live in Costa Rica. Actually, I was severely deficient in oxygen, severely anemic, and not thinking very well. As I was soon to learn, I was fast sliding into cachexia.

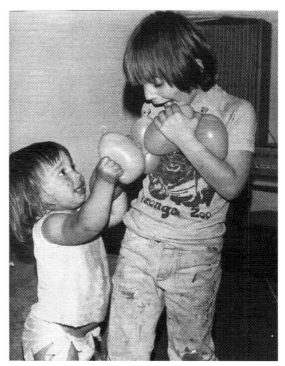

Chris' "babies", water balloons, kept "jumping" but Dmitri "rescued" them.

---Photo by Jen Kimberley

Juan agreed to keep my car in his parking area and drive it weekly for its health. We exchanged email addresses and with Dmitri's help, I stumbled out to the rental car. We left late April and drove back up the alarming mountain road to San Jose.

Before going to the airport next day, we got up early and went to my bank to finish the money transfer we had started at my local branch in Puerto Viejo, me limping along slowly, holding onto Dmitri. We allowed two hours for this at the branch closest to the airport, planning to reach the airport two hours before flight departure.

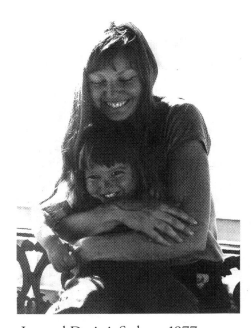

Jen and Dmitri, Sydney, 1977

---Photo by Unknown

We found someone who spoke enough English to show us to the right group of tellers for an international transfer. One of them spoke good English, as we could hear, and we asked to see him. No. We had to see the woman next to him who spoke no English at all. Someone gave her a brief explanation of what I needed and she started poking around on the computer. She stopped periodically, got up, and consulted with somebody in the back. She peered at a lot of papers, pecked on the keyboard, and ignored us entirely.

There was a clock on the wall and we watched it creeping towards our departure time. Our attempts to speak with the teller who spoke English were brushed away, as he was too busy. Dmitri nabbed the original man who spoke some English and explained that our plane was leaving in two hours, and could this woman please hurry up. The procedure was already started and she only had to finish it.

The man mumbled something in Spanish and disappeared. I kept drooping over the woman's desk, drifting into sleep. The time for our plane departure came and went and we sat there for a total of five hours. It turned out that the woman was new and timid and had to check each step with someone else. Eventually I discovered that she had decided something was wrong with how I'd been set up as a customer 18 months previously and she scrapped it, entered me as a new bank customer and re-created my entire bank record. I'd opened this account when I'd bought the land. In Arizona later, I discovered that I had no internet access, something I had carefully obtained back in Puerto Viejo but she had eliminated it.

So we missed our plane and had to get a hotel room where Dmitri arranged for another flight the next day. One of the great things about Dmitri is how he can handle problems. He stays calm and rational whereas I tend to get upset and useless.

The next day, we arrived early at the airport and the plane left punctually. But now we were a day late and thanks to that bank teller who scrapped my internet access, I was soon to be many dollars short. My appointment at the clinic was for Friday morning. We wouldn't be there till Friday night.

Energy Work #2: Being in Your Own Space

Learning to ground from the first chakra and be in your own space is the beginning of spiritual detoxification. It's central to happiness. We can feel happy for many reasons – loving parents, a loving marriage, success at work, a rising income, travel adventures – but these kinds of happiness rely on someone else. If your marriage breaks up, you lose your job, or get demoted to lower pay, your happiness will fly out the window.

Happiness that depends on nobody else is only obtainable from spiritual detoxification, from being yourself and living in your own space. Some would mention God at this point but that's a huge topic outside the confines of this Saga. As spirits living in bodies, we have the choice of whether to be in our bodies or out of them. Or partly in and partly out. Most of us are unaware of whether we're in or out although Mindfulness has become more popular in recent years – more people are more mindful of Mindfulness.

At the Institute in California that taught how to work with energy, one of the first things we learned along with Grounding was Center of Head. That's a straightforward name that means what it says – behind the eyes and between the ears. It's the Sixth Chakra of the seven main chakras we have in the body and it provides us with mental vision.

"Oh, I see what you mean."

"I don't see any difference between your goals and mine."

"Yep, I can just see that happening as you talk about it."

It's also called the Third Eye as it provides us with clairvoyance when we clean it out and still the rational mind, the chatter of the left brain. We may not have conscious clairvoyance, but we all have some degree of wordless vision – brief pictures or images that flash through our awareness and are often dismissed so quickly that we forget we had them.

For a long time I had trouble finding the center of my head. One day I saw that I'd learned early in life to live forward, in front of my body, trying hard to please my mother.

I was using effort. Very uncomfortable; but to me it was as familiar and unavoidable as putting one foot forward at a time to walk. To change the habit and live in my own body and Center of Head meant clearing out many layers of pain, invalidation, grief, and anger. I set to work on it and with periodic help over the years, I now can find Center of Head each time I wander out of it. But I do forget at times and get excited about something and get out in front of myself. Then I might need quiet time later to reassemble myself, heart and head.

It's tiring to live outside the body. If you suffer from chronic fatigue, have a look at whether you spend a lot of time outside yourself. Many generous givers do this, attending to other people's needs and forgetting their own.

Also, when we spend time outside the body, we leave it vulnerable to energy from foreign sources.

- A cancer patient tends to draw attention and energy from many people, not all of it well-meant. If your doctor sees you as someone whose days are numbered, he will likely throw that picture at you unconsciously, even if he or she doesn't outright say so. People who might have been envious of you for some time, or jealous, without you even knowing, might now throw a similar picture: "You're done for, buddy, Ha!"

We all tend to live chronically muddled up with each other energy-wise and in my view, that's a big reason why conflict develops, marriages fail and children rebel or misbehave. We become spiritually toxic from foreign energy mucking up our own energy flow. By "foreign" I mean it belongs to someone else. In their space it would be comfortable and productive but if it gets in your space, it doesn't fit; it feels uncomfortable, though you might be so accustomed to its presence that you don't notice it. OPE, Other People's Energy, is an ongoing issue for most of us, even highly trained and proficient energy workers, teachers of energy work, directors of energy work schools.

If we only knew, we're all happier in our own space and if someone else is in there with us, even someone we love, it's uncomfortable and in the longer haul, destructive. And looking at it in the other direction, if we are pushing our energy into other people's spaces, it's not then available to us; repeatedly doing this leaves us with noticeably less energy, and low energy is a contributing cause of disease.

In fact, all disease begins as energy. When your own energy is reduced, foreign energy will fill the gaps and now disease is gradually developing. I believe one reason why breast cancer is so prevalent is that our culture puts constant focus on women's breasts, encouraging male attention and energy invasion, and many women play into that.

Three Exercises on Center of Head

1. While going about daily activities, notice the distance between you in your head and the computer screen or roomful of children or vacuum cleaner – whatever your attention is focused on. Allow yourself to be separate from your focus. Don't become what you're doing; just let yourself do it and watch from the center of your head.

2. When sitting quietly somewhere, ground yourself and then focus your eyes on something nearby; then switch focus to something else and notice the difference in distances from you in the center of your head. Change focus again. Look out a window at a tree, for instance, then at a pen on your desk, then at your hands in your lap. It's like exercising a "seeing muscle". Awareness moves with the eyes but you stay still in yourself.

3. Sitting quietly grounded and in the center of your head, or as near to it as you can get, be aware of the room you're in, of the building, of the plot of land it's on, of the neighboring buildings and the streets. Start close and gradually expand. Let your awareness encompass 360 degrees, including any sounds and activities. Notice that none of it is You. If you hear a child crying or a dog whimpering, for example, don't get involved. Stay back in your own space. Notice how your body reacts but don't merge with that other energy.

When you are finished, fill yourself up with your gold sun. Sessions like this help with spiritual detoxing and detoxing promotes calm and happiness.

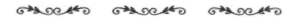

Memorandum

- ✓ A sugary diet contributes to cancer development;
- ✓ Low oxygen in the body cells also contributes to cancer development, a fact discovered by Dr. Otto Warburg in the 1920s;
- ✓ Dr. Johanna Budwig discovered Omega 3 and Omega 6 fatty acids and found that oils high in those are also highest in oxygen;
- ✓ Dr. Budwig devised a blend of cottage cheese and flaxseed oil that delivers oxygen to body cells, protecting them from becoming cancerous, and if they're already cancerous, helping them revert to normalcy;
- ✓ Dr. Max Gerson developed an effective cancer protocol based on a high-quality diet, detoxification, and immune system strengthening. It is still used by many today.
- ✓
- ✓
- ✓

Chapter 3: Emergency IV Care

"OK, found an apartment, Mum."

It was Saturday and we'd crashed into this Phoenix hotel room last night after the flight from San Jose. I grinned weakly at him from the hotel bed. I'd known he would. I needed one just a short walk from the clinic and I was trusting that my balance would improve so I could walk back and forth pushing a walker. Dmitri's employer had given him three weeks off and good man that he is, he was giving them to his Mum in her emergency. I was as dependent on him as a small child.

"It's temporary for one week because the one I want for you won't be vacant till then."

My anemic brain was following along but not able to frame a question. Dmitri sat on my bed and fluffed the blanket over me.

"We can move in on Monday. It's a one-bedroom apartment, furnished. In a complex, not a huge one, but in a nice area and just three blocks from the clinic. Big old trees. Not much traffic. I think you'll like it.

"Thanks, dear guy."

"I can sleep on the living room floor. I'll go to Walmart or somewhere and get an air mattress. Better than the couch. It has towels and saucepans and plates. The building manager has an office nearby in case you need anything."

He got up and went into the bathroom. I felt cozy and safe and started drifting into sleep again but I heard him get something from his duffel bag and say, "I'll be back soon and we can figure out some dinner," and the door closed softly.

It was dark when he returned. I heard him open and close the door, cross the room and close the curtains, and then say,

"You awake, Mum?"

I rolled on to my back. "Yes."

"Walmart has everything." He sat on the bed. "I got myself a pillow and sheets and I got you a heating pad and a bunch of little things. He pulled stuff out of the shopping bags and spread them on the bed. "Figured you'd need these things." Stapler, postits, pens, pad of paper, black Sharpie, sticky tape, paper clips.

"Thank you, Meech. I think I will need these."

"On Monday after you're finished at the clinic, we can unpack in the apartment and see what else we need."

We drove to the clinic on Monday morning. I had no appointment but the staff kindly squeezed me in. Dmitri had called on Saturday to apologize for missing our appointment. The clinic is in a nicely-built old house with large windows and doorways. You enter to a small receptionist room and from there go to a central room with a large table in the middle, large glass-fronted cabinet on the right, and easy chairs with side tables. The center table is for the morning snack (that day it was chocolate-coated kale crisped up in a dehydrator), everyone's daily jars of vegetable juice, and the boxed lunches and dinners brought from the clinic kitchen. The cabinet contains books and supplements.

The receptionist introduced us to a nurse, who took us to one of the three treatment rooms off the central room. Each is lined with recliners and all but one of them contained a patient receiving an IV treatment. I was settled into that empty one and the nurse took my vitals. Dmitri stayed with me and talked to the nurse, filling her in on my situation.

My New Patient Talk

I don't recall much about those first few days, but I do recall the New Patient Talk from Dr. Thomas Lodi, the founder and director. Dr. Lodi is an energetic man with a passion for teaching people how to stop creating their cancer. He spends about two hours with each new patient at Oasis giving them this talk.

It was impressive and persuasive and took place in his office, door closed, Dmitri present, Dr. Lodi behind his desk.

"Jen, do you know that wild animals that never come in contact with humans or our poisons die from three causes only: starvation, trauma, or old age. Why is that?"

I blinked, seeing a bony lion prowling around in search of some poor little deer. Dr. Lodi didn't wait for an answer.

"Why don't they get heart attacks, cancer, ulcers, arthritis or strokes? How come hundreds of animals can drink from the same watering hole without getting sick and we drink bottled water and we're all sick? Did Nature design us to be inferior to every other creature? Of course not! Our problem is that we've turned away from Nature, from God. They're the same thing, God and Nature. We think we're different from everything else living on this planet. We're delusional and think that Nature's rules don't apply to us.

"We have no clue about what our best functioning is because we've been so distant from it for so long. There are mountain people in Peru and in the Hunza valley who live well over 100 years and at that age are still climbing steep mountains daily with no effort. Most of us in the Western world who live to 90 or so are wearing diapers and nodding off in some nursing home hallway with tubes in our noses."

My past days as a nurse in a "convalescent" hospital floated before my eyes. I liked his humor and his obvious sincerity and since he was looking directly at me with his dark eyes blazing, I paid attention.

"Where is our human niche on this planet? If we weren't encultured to the point of being hybrid-mutants, we'd be in the tropics. Anthropologists say the first humans appeared in Africa -- a very tropical environment. The bible puts us in a green garden with lots of fruits and vegetables and seeds. It's thought to have been Mesopotamia, "the land between two rivers", which is now Iraq. Under that present-day desert is lots of oil, created by millions of fossilized plants under pressure with bacteria for eons. Living in the tropics, we ate what nature abundantly grew for us.

"But we left our paradise niche and wandered to other environments, adapting to ice, desert, wind, and high elevations, and now look at what people eat: Eskimos eating raw whale blubber; Thai people munching beetles, grasshoppers, and scorpions; live monkey brain is a delicacy in Malaysia; and in Italy, a popular cheese called Cazu Marzu is served swarming with maggots. I conclude from all of this that people will eat anything a cockroach will eat, including the cockroach – and then proudly defend it."

I laughed at these disgusting pictures.

"What's the difference between hunger and appetite?" He paused, gazing at me, but I had no answer.

"You know the saying, 'You have to acquire a taste for it'? Well, don't! That will override your hunger instinct and replace it with an appetite. Your reluctance to eat Wonder bread and Velveeta comes from your body's wisdom. Donuts and coffee feed an appetite, not your hunger. People develop appetites for liquor, narcotics, maggots and cigarettes, not to mention Big Gulps, hot dogs, and Twinkies. Feed your hunger, not your appetites!"

Dr. Lodi contrasted cats and dogs (lions, leopards, hyenas, jackals etc.) with all other mammals. Cats and dogs have jaws that move only vertically (not sideways or forwards), long tongues, acidic saliva, sharp back teeth, no cheeks or lips, and a relatively short and internally smooth digestive tract.

"And how do they eat?" he demanded. "Well, cats chase an animal and break its neck with their jaws. With their teeth, they tear open its abdomen and eat the liver, kidneys, rectum, the intestines with partially digested materials, the lungs, and the heart. They drink the blood and chew the bones and eyeballs. If they save anything for the vultures, it's what we call *steak*."

I couldn't disagree with any of this, being a lifelong cat owner and recipient of loving gifts in the form of mangled bird carcasses.

"Cats are called carnivores. Now Jen, I'm pretty sure that if a family member or friend of yours brought a chicken here this evening, you would not rip its head off and eat it alive. You and I are not carnivores."

I goggled at him, not knowing whether to laugh or puke, and not daring to look at Dmitri sitting to my right.

"Then there are the dogs. They're scavengers. They have digestive systems similar to the cats but like us humans, they prefer to eat the corpse. However, dogs listen to their instinct which tells them not to eat any corpse over three days old – it's now food for insects, bacteria and fungi. But what do we humans do? We know that a stiff corpse with rigor mortis will break our teeth, so we hang it upside down for four to fourteen days and call the decay "aging". We scoop out the pus and maggots and send the remains to the butcher. The butcher slices the corpse into pieces, packages them and puts them on display at the supermarket.

"We then buy these decayed remains of corpses but at home, we find them unappetizing as is. The oven or frying pan helps; then salt, pepper and a sauce or ketchup have us eating dinner happily. We humans do **not** eat the food of carnivores. Nor the food of scavengers. We eat the food of maggots."*

Well, I'm sure you get the drift here. He was persuading me to be a vegetarian, and as I found very soon, he advocates a raw vegan diet, not only for cancer patients, but for anyone who wants to live long and prosper. I met one of his kids later, who had been raised on a raw vegan diet. He was a tall, strapping young man, clearly not deficient in protein, which is one of the concerns meat-eaters have about a vegan diet. Dr. Lodi's talk went on to cover how we create cancer for ourselves and how no treatment will work unless we change the conditions that gave rise to cancer in the first place.

Getting Started With IV Treatments

An Oasis of Healing is not a live-in facility although relatives and friends of any age are welcome to be with patients any time. It has two buildings – the main one, which Dmitri and I were in for this New Patient talk, and another around the corner called the Lifestyle building. Like the main building, it's also a gracious old house with beautiful woodwork and large doors and windows, plus an enormous yard. It contains the raw vegan kitchen, a classroom for "cooking" classes, a room with tables and chairs for eating or socializing, and a room for Lymphatic Drainage treatments. At the bottom of the yard is a huge garage with an area for PEMF treatments (Pulsed Electro-magnetic Frequencies), a trampoline for "rebounding", and an infrared sauna.

Dr. Lodi's approach is to detoxify the body from its years-old or decades-old debris, strengthen the immune system, and gently reduce the cancer to zero by targeting it with a form of chemotherapy called Insulin Potentiation Therapy. As he often reminds us, he doesn't cure cancer at all – the body cures itself when it's freed from the heavy metals, intestinal garbage, and daily living stress (mental, emotional, and physical). First and foremost, Dr. Lodi is an M.D but is also licensed as a homeopathic physician and certified in nutrition. So he brings knowledge from all these fields.

---

* This partial reproduction of Dr. Lodi's New Patient Talk comes with his permission both from my memory and from my copy of a short book he was writing that I was editing while living in Thailand the following year (2013).

Dmitri stayed with me for two weeks in Arizona. He bought me a good walker and for the two weeks he stayed, he pushed me to and from the clinic in that walker, as I couldn't push it myself yet. While I was receiving IV treatments, he went shopping and bought many more supplies I'd need such as batteries, scissors, colored markers, a weekly pill box for my many new supplements, a magnifying glass to read their labels, and graph paper to chart my blood counts. He had a phone installed and an internet connection for my laptop.

On the Monday we'd arrived at the clinic, I'd been put on oxygen 24/7 so Dmitri arranged for the tanks and tubes at the apartment and a small portable tank. After two weeks on oxygen (and with other treatments I'll get to shortly), I was able to push the walker myself. It had a bag under the seat so I could take books about cancer home to read. When Dmitri left two weeks later, I felt like weeping, not just because he was leaving, but also in gratitude for his saving me from a solitary death in Costa Rica and getting me into a viable situation. We stayed in email touch as always.

Two PICC Lines

Because my leukemia was severe (it had gone into its acute phase preparatory to escorting me out of this world), I was going to need weeks or months of treatment including many IV treatments, and many blood tests to assess my progress. So rather than have me stuck with a needle each time, Dr. Lodi sent me to a local hospital for a PICC line -- a Peripherally Inserted Central Catheter. It's a thin flexible tube that's inserted into a peripheral vein and extended further into a deeper vein. It remains there as long as you need IV treatments (up to one year, though it's usually a matter of weeks). As well as avoiding repeated needle insertions, a PICC line delivers medications deeper into the body than a typical IV line does.

The insertion is done by a specially-trained nurse. Mine was inserted into the left lower arm and the tip was positioned in the Superior Vena Cava, a large chest vein that brings venous (waste-carrying) blood to the heart so it can be pumped into the lungs and acquire a fresh load of oxygen in exchange for its waste load which we then breathe out as carbon dioxide. A dressing was secured over the insertion point to prevent the line from moving and all my IV treatments were done through the end protruding from my arm.

This all worked well for a few weeks but then I developed a blood clot in the PICC line. This obstructed it, blocking medications, and also posed the danger that the clot could detach and travel in the blood. If it were to enter the heart or brain, I would suffer a heart attack or stroke. So it was removed and a second one was inserted into my other arm. This time, a radiologist came to the clinic with equipment and performed the insertion both for me and for several other patients, following up with an X-ray to confirm that its position was correct. Once more, it worked well for a few weeks but then developed a blood clot and had to be removed.

These clots were not inevitable, but since I had CML they were not surprising. Chronic Myeloid Leukemia features increased platelets, low red cells and increased dysfunctional white cells. Platelets are necessary for clotting and my platelet count was dangerously high both when I arrived at the clinic and later on. At that later time, I went to a hospital for Platelet Pheresis (see p. 52).

IV Port Inserted

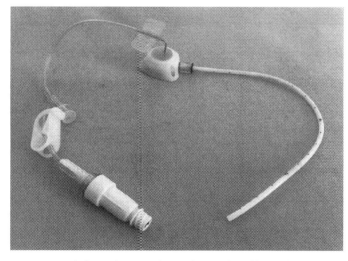

IV port. The tube on the right trails off inside a vein and has tiny holes and its open tip for medication to enter the blood. The needle (top) is inserted through the skin into the port and the fitting in the left foreground connects to the IV line.

---Photo by Jen Kimberley

Apparently, PICC lines were not for me, though they were worth trying, being simpler and less expensive than the alternative. But I needed the alternative and that was an IV Port. An IV port (also called portal meaning "entry point") is a little device about three-quarters of an inch wide and half-an-inch high, with a narrow, flexible catheter attached. Insertion is a surgical procedure done with local anesthetic in a hospital. Through a small incision, the port is inserted into the chest just inferior to (south of) the collar bone and creates a bump beneath your skin. It is not inside a vein – the catheter running from it is inserted into a vein with its end trailing off inside that vein to deliver IV medications. As with the PICC lines, the vein used was the superior vena cava. The port's top surface is a tough silicon that holds up for hundreds of needle pricks.

When the port is closed, as mine was over the weekends, the needle (top of photo, with blue wings) is removed and inserted into the other end of its short tube where there's a silicon surface like the top of the port itself (center left in photo). The other end (lower left), when not connected to any IV line, just dangles against your chest. Paper tape covered with waterproof plastic keeps the outside pieces in place. Inserting the needle into the two silicon surfaces requires a fair amount of pressure, as does removing it.

Each Monday morning, the nurse on duty would open access to my port by pulling the needle from the silicon end of its tube and piercing it through the chest skin into the silicon port surface. She would then suction out a little blood through that needle to make sure the internal catheter was clear and then flush it out with some saline solution (purified water with the same salinity – salt content – as the body's fluids). Then she would begin the first IV treatment by attaching the IV line to the dangling end that connected to the needle's tube.

During each week, when each IV treatment was finished, the nurse would detach the IV line from the port's dangling end and tape the port's external tubing to the chest skin, leaving the needle inserted into the port.

So that one needle prick on Monday mornings was the only one I had to have each week. I was glad to have this port and it remained in place until March 2013, after I had gone to Thailand.

Insulin Potentiation Therapy

This was one of the first treatments I had at the clinic, before the port was installed. It's a way of administering low-dose chemotherapy. Feeling as weak and ill as I did, I wondered why I wasn't offered super high dose chemo, but soon I learned that IPT is a sly treatment that sneaks up on cancer cells rather than bashing them blindly.

"Jen," said Heidi, the nurse in charge on my first day, "Please don't eat anything tomorrow morning. We need you to have an empty stomach for the first IV treatment."

Being still very anemic and lacking in oxygen, I nodded vaguely. I could hear her OK but I lacked the energy to discuss or enquire. I knew the phrase from my short career as a nurse years ago -- "NPO After Midnight" – "nil per os", as the ancient Romans would have said; "nothing by mouth". That is standard procedure before any surgery as no nurse or surgeon wants the patient to react to anesthesia by throwing up and ruining their sterile field. So after roughly midnight, no food, though you can drink any amount of water. IPT is not surgery – the reason for my NPO, as I soon learned, was to have my blood sugar low. Blood sugar is glucose that results from food being digested.

So next morning, I arrived with my stomach growling and got settled in one of the recliners ranged around the walls. Most of them were occupied, with Annette, the nursing assistant hopping from one patient to the next taking their vitals.

"Good morning, Jen," she said in passing. "I'll be with you in a minute. Would you like a blanket?" She was a slim, energetic young woman and I learned later that she was supporting two young children with this busy job.

I did want a blanket but she was gone. I was pretty sure she'd bring one when she returned and she did. She also brought two icy-cold mittens, two similar booties, and a freezing cold beanie.

"Put these on, Jen. They'll protect you from nerve damage potentially caused by the chemo drugs."

Meanwhile, Heidi arrived with an IV pole and a glass of something that she placed on my side table.

"Apple juice. Don't drink it yet. We'll give you a sweet snack too, for later."

Using my PICC line, she set up an IV saline drip.

"This saline will keep you hydrated while we do this treatment." I nodded, feeling like curling up for a good nap. No such luck. Heidi took hold of my left ear and pierced it. I instinctively raised my hand for protection. She had taken a drop of blood.

"Just getting your blood glucose level Jen," she said, looking at a little device in her hand. "Seventy nine. That's good. Average is about 75 to 100."

"Hundred what?" I mumbled.

"Milligrams of glucose per deciliter of blood." Given this briskness and obvious familiarity with what she was doing, I felt I was in good hands, so I didn't worry about understanding everything. I figured I'd read about it online later. I'd been pleased to see all the books in that glass-front cabinet.

Next, Annette pushed a thermometer at my ear, placed a device on one finger to get my pulse rate, and took my blood pressure.

"Good numbers, Jen. Here's a blanket for you." She draped it nicely over my extended legs and handed me a pillow. "Take it easy girl. We'll get you perked up in no time." I gave her a little grin.

Next, Heidi returned with a tray full of syringes and inserted one into a tube that ran into the main tube bringing the saline from a bag on the IV pole.

"This is Toradol," she said, laying the now-empty syringe in her tray. "It's an anti-inflammatory. And this one —" as she picked up another syringe, "is insulin."

"I don't have diabetes," I objected feebly.

"No. But we want your blood sugar to get low, so we're going to wait a few minutes now and I'll check it every so often." I got more comfortable with the blanket and pillow and closed my eyes. The room was warm from sunshine and I listened to everyone's voices without noticing what they were saying. I thought about Dmitri in the rental car, out shopping for stuff I'd need soon. We were still in the first apartment but about to get the second one. Someone had already booked the first one for a certain date and the occupant of the second one was about to leave. These were both apartments kept in reserve for Oasis cancer patients. What a capable and loving person Dmitri is. I felt warm and grateful and safe.

Soon Heidi was back, poking my ear lobe again. Apparently my glucose level wasn't low enough yet, because she left; then returned with another tray of syringes. Annette placed something on my side table.

"Here's your Sweet Treat, Jen." I perked up and found that it was chocolate pudding.

"Don't eat it till we tell you. It's from the kitchen and they make it with avocado." Well, that was intriguing – a combination of two of my favorite foods. I felt I was beginning to like this IPT treatment. Heidi poked my ear again.

"Good, Jen, it's down to 51 from 79. That's close enough to 60% of the starting point." I was glad to hear this because I was now feeling shaky and even more drowsy than when I'd arrived.

"Now your cancer cells are hungry for sugar and their membrane receptors are wide open for it."

She then got busy with syringes and in quick succession emptied four of them into the IV line.

"There. Now we're finished. I'll just give you this last one. It's dextrose, a sugar. We want to get your blood sugar level up to normal now. So go ahead and drink your apple juice and enjoy your pudding." She gathered up her empty syringes, alcohol wipes and whatnot and disappeared into the nurses' room. The pudding was super delicious and I resolved to get the recipe from the kitchen people.

IPT was done once a week on average, giving the body time to recover in between from any Die-Off (Herxheimer reaction) and a chance to detoxify the chemo since even low dose chemo is cumulative. The dead cancer and other cells had to be excreted to ready the body for more of them. I had IPT a total of 31 times during the eight months I was a patient at this cancer clinic. The ten percent (even five percent) dose saves you from the nausea and pain caused by full chemo. Supposedly it also keeps your hair from falling out, which happens with full chemo because those poison drugs are indiscriminate and besides killing cancer cells, also kill all fast-dividing cells such as hair follicles and protective gut bacteria.

However, most of my hair did fall out, leaving me with a sparse ring of hair as if I had my Dad's male pattern baldness. Another woman I talked with also complained about hair loss but her hair was much thicker than mine and she had no baldness. However, IPT did not give me any discomfort other than perhaps some extra fatigue, and for the baldness I was happy to buy a couple of hats. I've often wished hats were more fashionable. In supermarkets, whenever I notice a magazine on the rack with text or photos of the British royalty, I browse it – to look at the hats as much as their new babies. The big annual Ascot event is especially fruitful of extraordinary hats. (Continued on p. 49)

More About IPT

The term Potentiation states the procedure: insulin potentiates the chemotherapy drugs (makes them more potent) so that the ten percent dose is more powerful than it would otherwise be. Yet because it's only a ten percent dose, it gives only mild side effects, if any. The pancreas creates insulin, a hormone that regulates blood glucose (sugar) levels, keeping them steady. The IPT injection of extra insulin lowers blood glucose levels so that cancer cells are starved of it. Since cancer cells have many more insulin receptors on their membranes than normal cells, the injected insulin binds to them more quickly, making the membranes more permeable.

This creates the "therapeutic moment" when the chemotherapy drugs can enter the cancer cells at a much faster rate. Normally, the insulin acts like a door key for glucose, allowing the cell to receive glucose molecules; but in IPT, it is chemotherapy drugs they receive instead. Because of the extra insulin and extra insulin receptors, the cancer cells receive a much higher percentage of the drugs than normal cells and this is why IPT has diminished side effects yet achieves the intracellular concentrations of high dose chemotherapy treatments.

In the early days of IPT, the patient was given so much insulin that it produced an insulin coma. That is not done now. Enough is given to lower blood sugar to about 60% of its initial level, and the chemotherapy drugs are then given quickly, in that "therapeutic moment", followed by dextrose and sweet food and drink to restore normal blood sugar levels.

IPT has been used since 1930 when a family of three doctors devised it in Tijuana. In the three generations that they used it, there was never a negative outcome.

All the cancer drugs used in IPT have been approved by the American FDA (Food and Drug Administration). However medical students are not taught to use them in this IPT way and they regard IPT as an "unproven" treatment. Some conventional oncologists do administer low-dose chemotherapy but not with insulin.

IPT is an effective way to deliver chemotherapy; it is much less expensive than standard chemotherapy and requires far less of the drugs. In America, the state governments decide whether IPT can be administered, so if it is banned in your state, research other states.

A Blood Transfusion

In our first two weeks at the clinic, each of us went on a juice fast – no meals for two weeks but any amount of green juice.

"You won't feel hungry," we were assured. Right. I'd never done any sort of fast so I didn't jump on this idea.

"At least, not after the first two or three days," was the amendment. OK. Usually willing to try something once, I drank three or four quarts a day for 11 days. And indeed, I wasn't hungry after a day or two, though I still hankered for a good "Denny's" breakfast of hash browns, bacon and two eggs sunny side up.

On the 11th of my 14 days, with severe anemia, I had to go for a blood transfusion. The hospital had a supply of all types of blood and would infuse me with matching blood.

Chronic myeloid leukemia (CML) affects the main categories of blood cells differently:

1. White cells increase in total number because more and more dysfunctional white cells are made in the bone marrow. That's the cancer characteristic: no Off button, whether it's tumor cells or bad white cells.

2. Platelets increase and this puts you at risk for a blood clot that could travel in the bloodstream to the brain (causing a stroke) or the heart (causing a heart attack);

3. Red cells decrease, causing anemia. The blood gets cluttered with dysfunctional white cells and hasn't room to accommodate enough reds. And reds clumped together are less able to carry oxygen to body cells because their oxygen receptors

are on their membrane, their outside skin. This is "coin roll blood" and I certainly had it, as I found later in Thailand.

I was admitted as an inpatient and put into a room by myself for an overnight stay. After a few hours of waiting, a nurse set up the IV pole with a bag of blood hanging on it and inserted a thin catheter into my port. It took three hours or so for it to slowly transfer to my bloodstream and by that time it was dinner hour. They gave me a huge binder containing menus.

"I'm on a juice fast," I told the nurse. Does the kitchen have any green juice? The supply I brought has run out."

She looked doubtful but bustled off and returned saying, "They have no green juice but they do have three little cans of tomato juice. They're little three-ounce cans."

That would clearly be inadequate for continuing my juice fast and with all this interruption of my routines, I was now hungry so I said,

"Could you bring them? I'll see if I can order something too." I decided to end my fast which was approaching its 14-day term anyway.

The big binder had many tabs: diabetic diet, low fat diet, gluten-free diet, dairy-free diet, liquid diet and so forth. I looked in vain for the anti-cancer diet. Not there. So I just drank those little cans of tomato juice, preservatives and all, and finally went to sleep. They wanted to monitor me after the transfusion so that's why I was there overnight. I slept pretty well and was discharged next day.

Stumbling Through Cachexia

A month or so after that blood transfusion, I had to get another one, as my blood was still in an emergency state. I have an image of my blood from a dark field microscope, captured by Dr. Palo in Thailand (Chapter 6) but its resolution is too low for print output. I'll post it at jenkimberley.com when that site is created. It illustrates coin roll blood – the red cells are immobile and clumped like piles of pennies instead of being separate and active. The dysfunctional white cells show up as bright white but smaller than normal white cells would be.

When I had arrived at the Oasis clinic, my CML had gone through its accelerating phase, the white cells rising moderately fast in Canada and (unbeknownst to me) more quickly in Costa Rica, and on my arrival in Arizona, was in its acute phase. Without the excellent care given to me, I would have died. That would have been the standard outcome of CML and I was just one year later than the predicted time of nine-and-a-half years. My diagnosis had been in November 2001 and my leukemia-caused stroke occurred in March 2012.

Leukemia patients with CML do not typically live beyond the acute phase because conventional care does not include nutritional improvement, strengthening one's immune system or detoxifying the patient to offset the effects of chemotherapy, radiation or surgery. So when the acute CML becomes more aggressive, crowding the blood with junk white cells, raising platelets to dangerous levels, and preventing red cells from bringing oxygen and nutrients to body cells, the body has little or no ability to survive.

During this whole period from about November 2011 (still in Canada) to August 2012 (four months into my integrative cancer care, I was in what's called "cachexia" (pronounced kakexia) – the body wasting away for lack of functioning blood. I had been losing weight in Costa Rica, which is why I said to Greg,

"Do you notice that these restaurant chairs are getting harder every day?"

My derriere cushion was disappearing but I didn't notice that. I was just puzzled as to why the chairs felt harder. In Arizona, I continued losing weight, dropping from about 138 pounds to 109 pounds. My muscles lost their (modest) bulk and strength and my appetite dwindled. However, it didn't dwindle to nothing, as it does typically, to where the patient can't or won't eat anything and thus becomes even weaker. The Oasis treatments were clearing toxins from my system and maintaining a certain level of nutrient absorption with the result that after about four months I started regaining weight slowly.

In my understanding, not many leukemia patients have lived through cachexia and now, in November 2019, I'm eight years past my expiration date. In Arizona, though I regained much health and strength, I did not recover from this leukemia and I still have it. There's something keeping it in place and it's up to me to discover what, and to remove that condition. For my current protocol, please see Chapter 10.

Platelet Pheresis

Back to the Arizona clinic. Unlike some other leukemias, Chronic Myeloid Leukemia features high platelet levels and a month or so after the second transfusion, my platelets were almost at a million per cc of blood. The normal range is 150,000 to 450,000 per cc of blood and mine had risen quickly to about 960,000. I could have sustained a fatal blood clot any time. So I was scheduled for a hospital treatment to physically remove platelets from the blood. This is a type of blood dialysis and was done in the hospital's dialysis unit. I was settled into a recliner with blankets and next to me was a large machine.

"Could you turn that machine so I can see what it's doing?" I asked the nurse. She was not able to turn it 90 degrees but I could now see it at a slant. There was a window and below it and connected up to it was a tangle of tubes running from various vials and interspersed with assorted knobs. This machine collected my blood from an IV line the nurse connected to my port, separated and kept lots of the platelets, and returned the remaining blood to me. I believe these machines are also used when people donate platelets for people with bleeding disorders. I think it took about two hours. After this procedure, my blood was closer to normal and I haven't needed any second pheresis.

However, CML being aggressive in its acute stage, my platelets did push their way up too high on several subsequent occasions and Dr. Lodi prescribed Lovenox. This is an anti-coagulant, a long-acting form of heparin. Platelets work in just the first part of the coagulation process so if they are kept close to their normal range, the clotting sequence does not get out of hand. I had a collection of small syringes to self-administer Lovenox each evening. In other words, every bedtime, I had to stick a needle into my belly. It was just sub-cutaneous however, not deep down into some vein I had to find, so the needle went diagonally below the top layer of skin and thus didn't cause bleeding.

Other IV Treatments

As the days and weeks floated by, I was also given an assortment of detoxification and immunity-strengthening treatments.

- Vitamin C, 50 grams – 45 times
- Vitamin B Complex – 47 times

- Minerals – 39 times

- Heavy Metal Chelation – 21 times. There was a Heavy Metal test early on that indicated I needed these treatments. I had high (but not dangerous) levels of Cadmium and Thallium and just behind those two were Lead and Mercury. Nine others were at "safe" levels.

- Ultraviolet Blood Irradiation – 8 times.

- Alpha Lipoic Acid – 51 times. This is a strong antioxidant that kills free radicals.

- Autohemotherapy (ozone blood treatment) – 21 times. A small amount of blood is removed from the body, exposed to ozone and then returned to you.

There were four or five other IV treatments given just two or three times when I was in especially bad shape.

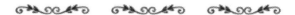

Memorandum

✓ If you consider a cancer clinic, look for one that offers powerful and beneficial treatments and research those treatments so you understand them.

✓ Cachexia can be the end of the line for a cancer patient but it doesn't have to be. Building your immunity up and removing poisons from the body enables you to start building your body's health such that cancer will be unsupported.

✓

✓

✓

Chapter 4: Non-IV Treatments

Colon Hydrotherapy

If I'd had my druthers, I would never have had this treatment. The idea of having someone insert a tube into the rectum and flush out the large intestine's contents with water was completely repugnant to me. But I was scheduled for it early on and in my dangerously poor health and chronically drowsy mental state (oxygen 24/7 was improving it but I had yet to go for any blood transfusions), I hadn't the energy to resist.

At my appointment time, I was sitting in the central room, just finished with one of the IV treatments. A tall woman emerged from the corridor leading from the central room to Dr. Lodi's office and several others.

"Jen? Jen Kimberley?"

She glanced round at the two or three others sitting nearby and her eyes came to rest on me.

"Hi, Jen. I'm Margaret.* Are you ready to do your first colonic treatment? You can bring the walker." She had a natural and warm smile. So I dragged myself up from the comfy chair, put my book under the walker seat, and trundled after her down the corridor. It went past two doctor's offices and she stopped outside Dr. Lodi's office where Dmitri and I had been given his New Patient Talk. The corridor was too narrow to park the walker there and still leave room for people to walk by, so Margaret helped me into the small bathroom and then parked my walker back in the central room folded up out of the way.

"Jen, you can put on one of these gowns," she said, pointing to a pile of them on a shelf. "Then just come on in and we'll get you comfortable on the bed."

The small bathroom had a folding door which she closed and I got myself into the hospital gown, a blue cotton garment that was visually familiar from my long ago nursing days but not familiar on me myself.

---

* Not her real name

When I made it the three yards into her colonics room, holding onto the walls, she helped me on to the bed, which was like a massage table with a white sheet and pillow and one of those soft hospital pads with a plastic backing.

Before I lay down, I looked at her machine. It was attached to the wall and had a transparent screen across the front, various knobs and controls front and top, and a long tube. Her calm and confident friendliness helped, but I still felt apprehensive and embarrassed. Margaret, to help me relax, gave me an essential oil to sniff. It did smell wonderful. Then she gave me two things to hold: a soft, squeezy ball for one hand and a rock for the other.

"If you squeeze both, they'll scramble your neurotransmitters," she explained. "You won't be so nervous."

I lay on my left side as requested, squeezing the balls hard, and Margaret began.

"This tube doesn't hurt, Jen. It's lubricated and I'll go slowly. You might feel a little bit uncomfortable but it's only temporary. You're in a perfect position – thank you." As she talked, she gently and deftly inserted the tube a short way.

She had some soft music playing that I would call musak. I asked if she had any other music.

"Yes, there's classical music, Louis Armstrong, Ella Fitzgerald …"

"Could you play some Ella?"

"Yes. Now, can you roll onto your back please? I can raise your head up if you like, so you can see what's happening." She propped the bed up so I could see both her and the machine. "How's that?"

"OK," I mumbled, pulling my hospital gown down as far as I could. She kindly arranged a large towel over me, then took the musak out of the CD player and soon Ella was filling the room with "Just one of those things, just one of those craaazy flings …" I hummed along in agreement.

"First we'll put some water in. You let me know when you feel full."

She turned a knob on the machine and soon I felt the water filling me up. It was a comfortable temperature. I kept my eyes on her hands as one re-arranged the curves of tube on the end of the bed and the other rested on the knob. The machine stopped after a minute or two and Margaret turned another knob. Suddenly the water in the tube turned brown and I saw objects travelling through behind the screen. They were various sizes and shapes. She could see things before I could because she was looking at the tube between me and the machine, and she made occasional comments.

"Those are small pieces of mucus. The colon's mucus lining is replaced about every three days. It gets the old pieces out so they don't create clutter."

She began to massage my belly with her left hand.

"Are you OK if I do this?"

"Yes." I figured she was dislodging stuck things.

She filled me up with water again and repeated the cycle. I began to marvel at all the things that had been in my intestines that didn't need to be there. I hadn't felt their presence.

"These are coming from the large intestine, is that right?"

"Yes, from the little nooks and crannies. The water dislodges them."

"Can we clean out the small intestine too?"

"Yes, but first we have to clear the large intestine and then the small one will have somewhere to discard its debris."

She repeated the inflow of water and outflow of debris several more times, massaging my belly, and then said,

"OK, would you like a quick coffee enema to finish things off?"

Enemas were another thing I'd resisted ever since I'd heard about them.

"It just takes five minutes. It's your decision. But I have coffee here in case you do want it. You have your own bucket – did you know that?" She pointed up to a small plastic bucket hanging above the foot of the bed and I saw that it was half full. "Coffee helps clean out the liver. It draws debris out of it."

I knew it was important to keep the liver functioning well. For the eight years I'd taken the Gleevec and Sprycel and the years on Bill Henderson's protocol, I'd eaten parsley every day, having read that it helps to detoxify the liver.

"OK, I'll try the coffee."

"Roll over on your left side again, Jen."

It took just a couple of minutes to empty the bucket.

"You're holding it well," she said. "You can stay there for five minutes or so. Let it soak in. I'll write some notes."

Then it was all over and I went to the bathroom. There was a small stool to rest your feet on, putting you in an optimum position for releasing. While I got dressed, Margaret fetched my walker.

"You did well! You get an A Plus. I can see you'll be my star performer!"

I grinned, still a bit uncomfortable but glad I'd started on a treatment I reluctantly admitted that I needed.

Margaret got me well started and I had that procedure two or three times a week for about eight months. She taught me to feel at home with it and she answered all my questions. (Narrative continues p. 64)

Mind Your Pees and Poos

The body has a multi-faceted excretory system consisting of:

- The kidneys • The bowel • The liver
- The skin • The lungs

Of those parts, the only one most of us routinely clean is the skin. Internal body cleansing is not so familiar to us as external cleansing, but the other excretory parts will benefit from periodic cleaning too:

Since the 19th century Industrial Revolution, our world has been getting more poisoned and more toxic to us and all living creatures. There are many books and websites that give details on the countless aspects of this, such as how food additives are toxic to our body systems, agricultural practices are damaging once-fertile soil; bees are disappearing from the planet; and environmental electro-magnetic frequencies such as from microwave ovens and WIFI damage our health.

So each day our bodies are bombarded with increasing numbers of toxins coming in too fast for our excretory systems to keep up with. Over the years, excess amounts build up and are stored in body fat or the liver; or they get mixed up with the nervous system, causing brain-related diseases, or they remain in the blood reducing its job performance in (a) bringing oxygen and nutrients to all body cells (arterial blood) and (b) carrying away cell waste products (venous blood).

For cancer (and all degenerative diseases), detoxification is the other side of the treatment coin. They go together in any successful approach. To focus only on putting things into the body and ignore getting things out is to pretty much guarantee that any improvement will be temporary. One thing we can do for ourselves is to look at what we excrete each day. Don't let yourself feel like some pervert. The contents of the bowl (and bowel) can tell us important things about our health status.

The Food's Journey

We have a small intestine and a large intestine:

- The small intestine is about one inch wide and 20 feet long;
- The large intestine (colon) is about three inches wide and five feet long.

The stomach partially digests our food and drink, breaking them down into proteins, fats, and sugars. This creates a loose, mushy substance called chyme. Stomach pH is about 3.5 because of its hydrochloric acid.

The chyme travels from the stomach into the small intestine where most of the nutrients are absorbed into the bloodstream as it moves along that 20-foot distance full of hairpin bends. To help digest the fats, bile is added to it from the liver and the pancreas sends enzymes. Intestinal pH is about 8.4, quite alkaline.

The small intestine connects to the colon on the right side of the body (from our own viewpoint) near the appendix. The colon circumnavigates the small intestine, ascending up the right side (Ascending Colon), across the top (Transverse Colon), and down the left side (Descending Colon).

When chyme enters the colon, water is absorbed, making it more compacted. Now it's known as "stool". The last part of the colon is the short rectum and it has nerves that detect the presence of stool and notify our brain that we need to defecate. The rectum makes a right-angle turn and its opening is called the anus.

When chyme travels too slowly through the intestines, we become constipated – stool ferments and gives off gas. When it travels too quickly, we have diarrhea. One of the reasons for eating well and exercising regularly is to pace the chyme, avoiding those two problems. A clogged and cluttered colon is the highway to disease.

What is Urine?

Our urinary system is an excretory system for the myriad substances that dissolve in water. The kidneys, at the back of the waist, are bean-shaped, and fist-sized. They make urine constantly and it trickles down to be stored in the bladder. It's an independent system, quietly doing its job while thousands of other events are happening in the body. Unlike the bowel, it is not part of the digestive system.

Urine is mostly water about 95%, and the rest is urea, uric acid, amino acids and electrolytes. We produce more if we drink more water and less when we're dehydrated. We also produce more if we ingest a diuretic, a substance that stimulates the kidneys. Coffee and alcohol are diuretics. The daily amount of urine can vary from about half a liter to two-and-a-half liters. An ongoing amount less than 30cc per hour is possibly kidney failure, a life-threatening condition. When the kidneys become diseased from toxic over-burdening, the person can go on kidney dialysis but that's a short-term life-extension.

Healthy urine is pale yellow and has a slight odor or none. Dark yellow urine, almost orange, indicates dehydration and gives off a much stronger odor. The yellow is due to a substance called urobilin or urochrome but some foods can override it and give you orange or reddish urine, e.g. beets, strawberries, carrots. (Remember too that urine contains toxins which are typically yellow. Think of aging and neglected fingernails: they're turning yellow. The skin of an aging person who has never detoxified also becomes yellowish as the skin stores toxins the overloaded liver can't accommodate. And cataracts in the eyes are yellow – toxins stored in the lens. An eye doctor can see that.)

What Can Stool Tell Us?

When you put aside the myriad details we know about our human bodies and consider the simple basics, it's evident that the human body is a long tube with arms and legs. The tube starts at the lips and ends at the anus. Parts of it run straight downwards and other parts are coiled or run sideways. What happens inside this tube enables and supports life in everything attached to the tube – that is, the rest of the body.

We love to talk about what we put in the top end of this tube but are typically reluctant to talk about what we expel from the lower end. That's probably because of the way we get potty-trained:

"Don't play with your poo!"

Which is good and necessary at the time, given that stool is full of bacteria and a small child doesn't yet find it repulsive. But we learn to turn our backs on it and thus, in adulthood, lose an opportunity of assessing our own health free of charge. So we have a bit of relearning to do if we want to keep good tabs on our health via stool monitoring.

Characteristics of Healthy Stool

- o About three-quarters water so not sticky or hard to clean off;
- o Well-formed, clearly shaped;
- o Soft and smooth with no particles or lumps;
- o Medium or light brown or green if you drink a lot of green juice;
- o Comes out in one long piece, possibly as long as 18 inches;
- o Between one and two inches in diameter;
- o Falls quietly into the bowl;
- o Has little to no odor.

If your stool requires pushing, has small hard lumps falling separately, has visible small particles, or a liquid consistency, then something needs to be done to correct it. If it is red, black or yellow in color, a visit to your doctor would be in order. Passing gas is normal when it is a small, quiet, and odorless event; but if you suffer from gas pains or explosive gas expulsion, something is up and should be attended to.

You can get informed opinions on your stool from a good colon hydrotherapist. A simple addition to the bathroom that will help with constipation is a footstool. Sitting with feet on a footstool puts you in the best posture for elimination.

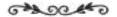

Coffee Enemas: How They Work

Instructions for how to do a coffee enema can be easily found online. It is an efficient way to detoxify the liver, blood and colon at the same time.

Upon entering the colon, the coffee liquid and its caffeine part company.

1. The coffee liquid fills the whole colon and by remaining there for 12 to 15 minutes, it loosens any stuck matter from crevices. A person who has for years eaten foods he or she has a sensitivity to and can't fully digest could have a lot of stuck matter, even to the point of its covering most of the colon's inner surfaces. If the colon is thus obstructed, stuck matter can back up into the small intestine and that reduces absorption of nutrients, eventually causing malnourishment. A saline enema would also help clear the gut of these accretions.

2. The coffee liquid's presence also stimulates peristalsis (gut movement that propels food along) and increases bile flow from the liver. That bile contains toxins, increased in amounts by the caffeine.

3. The caffeine is absorbed into tiny capillaries in the colon walls that flow into the hepatic portal vein, which carries venous blood loaded with waste products to the liver. When the caffeine arrives in the liver, it increases the liver's normal production of an enzyme called glutathione S-transferase by about 600%.

   The liver's incoming venous blood has gathered up free radicals from all over the body and brought them (with other waste products) to the liver to be disposed of. Glutathione S-transferase combines with them which disables them and the bile then carries them into the small intestine, and from there out of the body through the colon. The 600% increase in glutathione S-transferase vastly increases the liver's ability to process free radicals, and this cleans out the blood, also helping to prevent any liver overload.

During the 12 to 15 minutes the coffee is held in the colon, the blood circulates through the liver 4 to 5 times. Every 3 minutes it completes its journey through the body and brings another load of toxins and free radicals for disposal. So each coffee enema acts like a short blood dialysis treatment. Each also helps with eliminating intestinal parasites which are no longer a third world problem. Most people in Western countries now host them and you can get tests to specify which ones you have. If you have persistent digestive problems, a parasite test would be a smart move. For more on parasites, see Ch. 10.

How Ancient Are Enemas?

If you have been eating a lot of junk food, "baptism with water" can help undo that "sin". Below is text from the Dead Sea scrolls, the Essene Gospel of Peace, Bk 1, pp. 15 and 16, translated into English in 1937.

> "Think not that it is sufficient that the angel of water embrace you outwards only. I tell you truly, the uncleanness within is greater by much than the uncleanness without. And he who cleanses himself without, but within remains unclean, is like to tombs that outwards are painted fair, but are within full of all manner of horrible uncleannesses and abominations. So I tell you truly, suffer the angel of water to baptize you also within, that you may become free from all your past sins, and that within likewise you may become as pure as the river's foam sporting in the sunlight.
>
> "Seek, therefore, a large trailing gourd, having a stalk the length of a man; take out its inwards and fill it with water from the river which the sun has warmed. Hang it upon the branch of a tree, and kneel upon the ground before the angel of water, and suffer the end of the stalk of the trailing gourd to enter your hinder parts, that the water may flow through all your bowels. Afterwards rest kneeling on the ground before the angel of water and pray to the living God that he will forgive you all your past sins, and pray the angel of water that he will free your body from every uncleanness and disease. Then let the water run out from your body, that

it may carry away from within it all the unclean and evil-smelling things of Satan.

"And you shall see with your eyes and smell with your nose all the abominations, and uncleannesses which defiled the temple of your body; even all the sins which abode in your body, tormenting you with all manner of pains. I tell you truly, baptism with water frees you from all of these. . . . And this holy baptizing by the angel of water is: Rebirth unto the new life. For your eyes shall henceforth see, and your ears shall hear. Sin no more, therefore, after your baptism, that the angels of air and of water may eternally abide in you and serve you evermore."

This is all true in my experience and so I includeth it here for your enjoyment and betterment. Turn not your mind away from it. ☺

Electro-Lymphatic Drainage

Lymphatic drainage was a new concept to me. Of course I knew that the human body has a lymph system with nodes and that it somehow connects to the bloodstream, but I'd never heard of any lymph treatments, nor did I know what lymph does in the body. So when I pushed my walker into Victoria's treatment room, I had little idea of what to expect.

Victoria was a soft-spoken person and her room had a peaceful atmosphere. It was in the back of the Lifestyle building, a short walk from the main Oasis building. I pushed my walker up the ramp at the front main entrance, through the classroom and kitchen, saying Hello to the chefs and along a short corridor. It's a large room with a nice wood floor and four big windows. In the middle was a massage table and around the walls a couple of chairs and a small cupboard.

"Welcome, Jen," Victoria said. "Nice to have you here. Have you had a lymphatic drainage treatment before?"

We talked a little and I learned that a full treatment would include the whole body. But I was interested in regaining my full balance and hearing so I said,

"Could you just work on my head? Might that help clear the capillaries in the brain that got blocked by my TIA? (That's Transient Ischemic Attack, Dr. Lodi's opinion of what had happened to me in Costa Rica.)

"Yes, perhaps it could. I'll be glad to focus on your head and neck if you like."

So I took off my shirt and shoes and lay down on my back and Victoria picked up the two hand pieces trailing from her machine. Lymph flows downwards in the head, face, and neck to the soft area superior to the collar bone. That's a collection area with larger lymph vessels. So Victoria started by moving the handpieces outwards along each side of the collar bone to clear that area. She used a gentle pressure, her glass hand pieces gliding pleasantly over my skin, and a repetitive motion like sweeping the kitchen floor – short strokes to get all the bits and pieces followed by longer strokes to move them along.

Then she treated my whole face in four sections:

1. Along beneath the jawbone and down, using repetitive motions to cover the whole neck area;

2. Along and above the jawline, then down to the collarbone area;

3. Along the cheekbones beneath the eyes and down to the collarbone;

4. Across the forehead from center to each temple and down the cheeks and sides of the head and neck to the collarbone.

Periodically she again cleared the collection area out to the left and right sides. It felt calm and organized, working from the bottom to the top of the whole treatment area, including the ears.

Sunlight through the big old trees made dappled shadows on the white window blinds and a murmur of voices drifted from the kitchen where lunch was being prepared. A couple of people walked past the windows headed for the big garage at the rear of the yard. I floated in a peaceful daze.

"How are you feeling, Jen?" came Victoria's voice.

"Good," I mumbled. "Don't stop."

She laughed but she did stop when the half-hour was up. I sat up and waited a moment for the world to stop bouncing (it rocks with each of my head movements), then put my shirt and shoes back on.

"Can we do this again?"

"You bet. I think you're supposed to have lymphatics twice a week."

Our Lymphatics Education

Victoria taught a Lymphatics class at one point. She gave us all a diagram of how the lymph channels run throughout the body and where the watersheds are. She mentioned that there's another way of doing lymphatic drainage which is to use a manual technique, a feather-light touch rather than her gentle pressure and organized movements. She said that while that was a well-proven technique for moving Lymphedema (swollen lymph areas), it would be less helpful for cancer patients than the Electro-Lymphatic Therapy.

She ordered brushes so we could all stimulate our lymph flow according to the technique she taught us. This is known as dry skin brushing and is most beneficial done before a shower or bath. That way, you can wash off any dead cells remaining on your skin. The brush has a long handle and you can use it to scrub your back in the shower. The term "dry skin brushing" often refers only to the skin and it is indeed a good way to keep your skin healthy because it stimulates blood flow and cleans the skin surface. But when you do it for lymphatic drainage, you need to follow the direction in which lymph flows and to first clear each collection area so lymph flowing to it has a place to go.

Some say that lymph brushing should all be done towards the heart because all lymph flows that way but Victoria explained that this is not quite true. It's true that you brush upwards on the legs and arms, but that's not because the lymph in your limbs is flowing to the heart. It's flowing to the appropriate drainage areas. There, it delivers its waste material to the deeper lymphatic system, flowing through lymph nodes for filtering, then connecting with the venous system. From the heart, venous blood flows to the lungs where it gives up its carbon dioxide (waste material from cell respiration) and picks up oxygen from our in-breaths. Now it's arterial blood and carries oxygen to the cells (and nutrients according to your diet).

As an example of dry skin brushing appropriate for lymph flow, visualize an invisible pair of lines extending from the thumb to the armpit and from the little finger up over the shoulder to the collarbone. They divide the arm vertically, creating a track along the top of the arm and a wider area beneath it. There are watersheds on each side of those lines.

- Brush the underside and sides of each arm from the thumb over the inside of the wrist and up to the armpit, being sure to include any sagging bits at the back of the upper arm. Brush to the top of the armpit.

- Brush the top side of each arm from the fingertips over the back of the hand in a straight line up over the shoulder to the collarbone.

The armpits and the collarbone area are like lakes and the arm's lymph vessels are like rivers draining into those lakes.

I had lymphatic drainage twice a week for about eight months.

(Narrative continued on p. 69)

More About Lymph

Like the blood, lymph moves through the body in a system of one-way vessels, but it has no heart pumping it along. A clear fluid much like blood in composition except it has no red cells, its job is waste removal, working as an auxiliary to the venous system. When it isn't in lymph areas (see below), it's called extracellular fluid, the name for all body fluids not inside cells.

Lymph flow depends on body movements, the contraction and relaxation of muscles, which nudge the lymph flow along in nearby channels. Activities like running, surfing and dancing will certainly do the job, but deep breathing and moderate exercise like walking are also adequate. It will become clogged if your lifestyle is too sedentary.

Lymph connects to venous blood through tiny capillaries all over the body. It gathers up waste materials from body cells and on the way to delivering them to venous blood for disposal by the body, it passes through lymph nodes where some of the waste products are filtered out. Lymph is part of the immune system, and uses lymphocytes (named from *cytus*, Latin for cell: white blood cells that work with lymph). Please see pp. 3-6 for more on blood cells. Lymphoma is cancer of the lymph system.

Parts of the Lymph System

Lymph nodes cluster in groups throughout the body. They become swollen when the lymph is too stagnant or when there is bacterial or viral invasion. Their main task is protecting the body. Lymphocytes working in lymph nodes are central to our immune system. Although they are a type of white blood cell, less than one percent of them are found in the blood at any given time because they are busy at work in lymph nodes. Hodgkin's disease involves lymph node enlargement in the neck area that spreads through the lymph system, including the spleen.

The **spleen** is on the left side (from the person's viewpoint) below the diaphragm, opposite the liver. It is a blood filter, removing old or abnormal cells – this is why a cancer doctor will palpate the spleen looking for enlargement caused by too many discarded cells stuck in there. The spleen also helps to make antibodies – blood proteins that latch onto foreign proteins, immobilizing them so white cells can dispose of them.

The **Thymus**, in the upper chest near the neck, is both a lymphatic organ and endocrine gland. It houses lymphocytes while they mature and grow into T-cells (Thymus cells), white blood cells that attack foreign particles.

The **tonsils** are pieces of lymph tissue at the back of the throat -- clusters of lymphocytes held together with fibers. There are three pairs of them, one pair being the **adenoids**. They're the security guards at this gate into the body, destroying germs and sending out chemicals to destroy them. Tonsils grow through childhood and slowly shrink later in life. Sometimes they become infected and swollen, potentially blocking the windpipe and can be removed in a tonsillectomy. It used to be thought that a series of throat infections meant the tonsils were defective and many children lost their tonsils to surgery. I remember this from third grade when, most of the time, there were one or more kids absent, getting their tonsils removed. But the medical world has a better understanding now of their function.

Peyer's Patches (named for their 17th century Swiss discoverer, Hans Conrad Peyer) are oval-shaped nodules, small thickened masses, on the wall of the ileum, the last section of the small intestine. We have 30 to 40 Peyer's Patches and they create about 70% of lymphocytes. They conduct immunity surveillance in the ileum, joining as it does to the colon, which opens to the outside world and is thus a channel for pathogens to enter the body. (This mirrors the security guard work done by tonsils and adenoids at the entry gate to our digestive system.) The Patches facilitate disposal of pathogens through the colon.

DIY Hydrotherapy for Lymph Flow

Hydrotherapy is the use of water to heal the body. For improved lymph flow, contrast hydrotherapy using hot and cold water is effective when done properly. At the end of your shower, switch the water from hot to cold and back, ending with cold. Find your maximum toleration and let that hot water flow over your face and body for about three minutes, bringing extra blood to the skin. Then switch to cold water – cool at first if cold is too shocking – and run that over your body for 30 seconds or so until the skin blanches. Don't go so cold that you start shivering. Do this at least three times for best results.

This procedure increases both blood and lymph flow, thus helping to clear out toxins and waste products from body cells. By clearing the lymph nodes, it helps the lymphocytes in their filtering work. As with most activities, the more you do this, the more you become familiar with it and the body will tolerate a wider range of temperatures. Remember to end with the cold water and then keep warm after the shower. In combination with dry skin brushing before the shower, this can be an effective way to promote detoxification.

Energy Work #3: Creating Your Own Life

Was I creating my own life in this period? I certainly didn't feel that I was. I could walk only with sturdy support from Dmitri and after he left, only pushing the walker. Sitting, I faded and drooped within minutes. Planning and remembering were skills of the past. Submerged in illness, I vaguely mused about where was my life going? and was it supposed to be going there? I did more or less keep myself grounded and in my own space out of habit and stayed out of Dmitri's space – at least he didn't complain about me getting in his space. He knows a fair bit about energy tools because as small boys, he and his brother sat in on some of my classes, on the floor next to me drawing pictures or lying under my chair. Now I felt that I was – not lying under his chair, but curled up in a little red wagon he was pulling along.

Probably all of us have been in a weakened position, whether from illness or financial disaster or emotional troubles, where we depend on someone to help us out of it. We often think that the world is at fault, life is going against us;

"If only wretched Jane hadn't done that, I wouldn't be in this situation!"

"If they hadn't laid me off none of this would have happened!"

"I don't know why I've gained all this weight! It just happened!"

"The other car collided with mine without warning me of its intentions."

"I had been shopping for plants all day and was on my way home. As I reached an intersection, a hedge sprang up, obscuring my vision. I did not see the other car."

"The telephone pole was approaching fast. I was attempting to swerve out of its path when it struck my front end."

---From an insurance company newsletter, early 1990s

Yet as unlikely as it seems, there is a sense in which we create our own situations, both happy and miserable ones. We aren't necessarily aware of doing it – we create happenings by being who we are, by making the decisions we make, by being habitually hopeful or habitually cynical, by mentally dismissing possibilities because of arbitrary convictions that they couldn't become real; or conversely, by expecting happy outcomes despite apparently negative circumstances. We draw energy levels into our lives that match the energy we habitually run in our bodies. This is an over-simplification because there are other factors such as karma but it will serve for now.

There's an energy technique for consciously creating your life, for influencing events such that your life flows where you want it to flow. It's called making a mock-up and is quick and simple to do. On planet Earth, our lives are tangled together so that other people's energy is mixed up with our own. It might boost our goals or it might undercut them but either way, it is not our own energy and its presence in our space obstructs our own energy flow.

That's not to say that it's always ill-intentioned; much of the time it's very well-meant and the person is trying to help. They just don't realize that they're putting their energy in your space and thus setting you back in some way. Most of us are seldom aware of what we're doing with our energy and we can sabotage ourselves as often as not.

Picture yourself as a painter. You have a painting in mind and you want it to come out as you envision it. So you sketch out the painting's composition – where the tree should go, how long the fencing should be, where the moon should be for the desired shadows. Maybe you mix a few colors to test their effect on the eye and on each other. It's like a dress rehearsal for a play: try on the costumes, practice the timing, get the stage movements and positions fixed.

As a mock-up example, let's say your birthday is coming up and you want a certain kind of day. You want a late start for sleeping in; lunch out with your friend who never has time to see you; an afternoon trip to a beach with your family and doggie and no cell phones or video games; and a party in the evening with bright lights and good food and dancing. If you're dismayed at this image of a birthday, never mind; just substitute the things you would want.

An upcoming birthday is just an example. What in your life would you like to influence to be the way you want it? Sit down where it's quiet and you won't be interrupted. Ground yourself and find the center of your head. Picture a rose in front of you and let it represent the event or situation you want to shape. Put in that rose all the qualities you'd like to have – timing, outcome, emotions, other people's participation – whatever is relevant. Ground the rose, running the energy cord to the center of the earth as we do for our own grounding.

Fill the rose with everything you want but keep your own energy out of it. This is a neutral exercise; once it's completed, the rose mock-up functions without your help or attention. If you stay neutral, it will fall into place neatly and naturally. You might not even remember that you made a mock-up. When you are finished, explode the rose and don't worry that you're destroying your own mock-up – you've created it by putting the pieces together of what you want, and in a grounded form, and as long as you leave it alone, it will materialize.

You can do this any time, as often as you like. Would it affect anyone else's desires for the same event or situation? No. From their standpoint, it will happen according to how they've anticipated it, whether consciously or unconsciously. Their thoughts and behavior will create it consonant with their world. For example, everyone present at a birthday party will experience it according to their own (conscious or unconscious) mock-ups and their own havingness levels. (For Havingness, see pp. 144-146)

People who are big givers tend to worry about how their own plans will affect others, but such worry can often be unnecessary given how we all create our own reality.

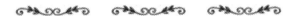

Memorandum

✓ Colon hydrotherapy is an important part of detoxifying the body.

✓ Paying attention to one's stool is a valuable part of monitoring one's health.

✓ Coffee enemas are a superb way of cleaning the blood and liver as well as the colon.

✓ Electro-Lymphatic Drainage helps keep the lymph moving so it can bring waste products from body cells to the venous blood.

✓ Our expectations of life play a huge role in determining our life flow. Changing your expectations can change the direction of your life.

✓

✓

✓

Chapter 5: A Diet to Discourage Cancer

The topic of what is the best anti-cancer diet is a huge one, controversial and evolving. I think that, as with treatments, one needs to approach it via testing and customizing. However, I stumbled through it blindly, giving it little thought beyond what tasted good until I found myself in Dr. Lodi's office listening to his New Patient Talk (see pp. 38-41). So on diet development, I started suddenly as a raw vegan.

The Clinic Kitchen

Two hard-working women ran the clinic kitchen, helped by a hard-working assistant. It was a small room with a very large wood table in the center and I had to walk through it each time I went for a Lymphatics treatment. Nobody minded; they just said Hello. There were always huge bowls on the table getting filled with salad vegetables. The dehydrators, essential appliances in a raw diet, were in the building's front room which was also a classroom, with two long tables for us to sit at and use the high speed blender or the spiroli or whatever was being taught that day. Carla, the chief "cook" gave these classes and I don't believe I missed any. I remember the first one: I fell asleep, head on table. Someone cited that to Dr. Lodi as evidence that I needed to get a blood transfusion to help with anemia.

Enzymes and the Raw Vegan Diet

Raw vegan food is a cuisine of its own. Although I'd never been a vegetarian before, let alone a vegan, such were the clinic meals that I didn't miss meat.

Enzymes are tiny proteins that facilitate things happening in the body. Each food from Nature (unlike factory-processed foods) contains enzymes appropriate for our digestion of that food. When food is heated over 104 degrees, some of these enzymes die and if the cooking temperature gets as high as 118 degrees, they all die. When you eat food with no enzymes, your body must provide the appropriate enzymes from its inborn storehouse. We have tens of trillions of enzymes in our body – not just for digestion, but for everything that happens in the body. We can't live or function without them. Each one specializes in a particular action or event, and is part of making that event happen, such as the enzyme Glutathione S-Transferase that binds with toxins in the liver, readying them for excretion (see p. 62).

Cooked food has none of the enzymes that were in the raw ingredients. As we get older, our inborn stock of digestive enzymes dwindles, which partly accounts for all the mid-life digestive problems – cooked food is not being fully digested (unless you take an enzyme supplement with meals). For raw vegan food preparation, the large tray-type dehydrators keep temperatures low enough to preserve all the enzymes.

A Man Aged 111: How Does He Eat?

One day Margaret said,

"Do you want to come to a potluck tomorrow? It's to celebrate someone's 111th birthday."

That got my attention. "You bet. Who is this person?"

"His name is Bernando and there's a group of people who do this potluck every year for him. It's all raw vegan."

So she picked me up the next morning and we drove to a private house. Many were already there and the welcoming hostess showed us to the back yard. I'd brought a fruit salad and Margaret had brought some avocado wraps. I'd never seen such a big trampoline! It took up half the large lawn area and served as the picnic table, loaded with colorful food arranged in two circles around its circumference. We found little spaces for our contributions and sat at one of the tables. People were chatting at many small tables and children were running around noisily. A large tortoise came to inspect our feet but apparently found them routine and moved leisurely on to the next pair. At our full table we all introduced ourselves. I looked around for an aged man in a wheelchair, white-haired and bent, with someone caring for him, but saw no such person.

Shortly, the hostess, Bev, appeared from the back door and announced that Bernando was here and he would give us a talk before we started lunch. Two men then appeared. One stepped forward and people started clapping. Bev grabbed some of the children dashing past him to quiet them down.

"Good afternoon, friends. Thank you for coming today. I love these annual feasts we have at Jim and Bev's house and I see today's banquet is rich and colorful as always."

He waved his walking stick at the trampoline with a big happy grin. He evidently didn't need that stick for support. He was slim and his posture was erect and easy. He was wearing summer slacks with an open neck shirt and a light jacket.

"Bev tells me we have some non-raw-vegans here today so I'd like to talk for a minute about diet and health.

"My father got me started. He was a doctor who also knew about herbs and he was a good teacher. He started when I was about five to teach me how to eat well and why it's so important. We ate a lot of fresh green salads and fresh fruit and nuts and seeds.

"I've often had fish so I haven't been a raw vegan. I've always liked salmon and sardines and fileted fish and lobster. They're all great sources of protein and many other important nutrients. Once a year I've been having lamb; that's been a special dish. But I've never had pork, beef, or chicken.

"I've always appreciated the raw vegan folks. That diet does make a lot of sense. We're all different and we each have to figure out what diet is best for our own body. We all know there are lots of diets out there and they're all advertised as the best diet for everyone, for different reasons.

"'What diet should I eat?' That's what people ask me when I give lectures. I tell them,

"'You go ahead and eat any diet that seems best for you. But make sure of two things. One, keep your colon clean; and two, keep your liver clean. If you do that, you'll be able to recover nicely from any minor health problem and you won't need any doctor visits.'"

"But as you all know, if we let those two organs get overworked or clogged up, we're in trouble. Lots of diseases can begin.

"I've seldom been sick and my mostly vegetable-based diet has always given me a nice light feeling, a happy stomach and the raw food goes in easily and comes out easily the other end, never have to worry about it. Fish is easy on the digestive system too. Moderation in all things, as the saying goes.

"As we all know, raw vegan food is a cuisine all to itself and I see a lot of you are very skilled at it. Friends, I'm very glad to see everyone here today and Jim is going to call out table numbers for everyone to get some good lunch without tripping over each other. Chow down, folks!"*

He waved his stick with a big smile for everyone and then hung it over the back of a chair kept vacant for him at a nearby table. Then he led his table mates to the trampoline.

"Table 9!" called Jim and everyone at our neighboring table got up to follow the others. We waited our turn which was slow in coming and I started hoping there'd still be something left for us. There must have been at least 80 or so people present. But when "Table 16" was called (numbers were random), the banquet still filled the trampoline perimeter with empty dishes pushed towards the center. Veggie burgers, rich avocado dishes, many kinds of nut or seed wraps overflowing with colorful veggie concoctions, nut or seed cheeses, huge bowls of green salad with choice of dressings, lush fruit salads, "baked" goods looking like any quality bakery counter but containing only raw ingredients, many puddings all decorated nicely with mint sprigs or chocolate designs that had been solidified in a fridge and were now starting to melt a bit.

The children had tables inside the house where Bev and some helpers kept them happy. Later a big birthday cake appeared, a chocolate cake with white frosting and "Happy 111th Birthday Bernando" in drizzled chocolate.**

Eating Out as a Raw Vegan

Many restaurants don't mind special requests and we can order a fresh salad at most of them. I take my own dressing. We can also take our own filtered water rather than accept what is often tap water or buy an overpriced bottle of "spring" water etc. Bottled water seems to have lost the public's trust these days. If I want to order a rare cup of coffee, I'll take a little tub of coconut creamer and a packet of Xylitol. One could also bring a tub of coconut butter for a baguette or toast and probably many other things, depending on your tastes and hopefully not offending the restaurant personnel. It's a matter of planning once you know what restaurant you'll be dining at.

---

* This talk given by Bernando is fictional, based on information at the website http://agelesslivemorestore.com/. My memory of his talk is not clear enough to use. That site sells the two books he wrote.

** Bernando had two more such birthday parties and in December 2015 he died at the age of 114, active and happy to the end.

Many Sundays a group of us went for lunch at a vegetarian restaurant that also served raw vegan food. I had my first veggie burgers and raw desserts and I was wowed. The desserts cabinet looked every bit as rich and scrumptious as any other and this is a desserts expert speaking. I sampled it each week – chocolate cheesecake, chocolate and strawberry cake, peach cobbler, even tiramisu – all made with raw ingredients and no eggs or dairy products. Some had stevia and some had sugar but Sunday was my day off from strict Raw Vegan so I didn't enquire about sweeteners when I decided on which dessert to order.

One Sunday Margaret and I went to a different restaurant from our usual one. As we walked in, admiring the pleasing wood floor and furniture, the owner, wearing her chef's cap, was finishing up with two other customers. While waiting, we looked at the menu posted on the wall behind the counter and I decided to have the sweet potato pie.

"Can I help you ladies?" came an authoritative voice. Margaret ordered an avocado dish and I said, "I'd like the sweet potato pie please."

"You can't have that."

"Oh. Are you sold out?"

"Oh no, I have several. But they're not for you."

I stared at her, puzzled. "Well I'm your customer and if you have it, I'd like to order it, OK?"

"No. You have cancer. I heard you two talking a minute ago. The sweet potato pie has too much sugar for you."

"You mean you add sugar to your recipes?"

"No. I mean sweet potatoes are too sweet for a cancer patient. I'd advise you to order the curried cucumber soup. It comes with your choice of extras, a salad, and crackers made with coconut flour and crushed almonds. Very tasty."

I paused, my slight annoyance giving way to a warming heart for this woman considering my needs, even though she was a bit abrupt about it.

"Well, thank you for looking out for my health. Not many people extend themselves to that and you're right that sugar is to be avoided. I have a strict regime six days a week but

Sunday lunch is my time to try new things and I've heard great reports of your menu here. I've never had a sweet potato pie before so I really would like to try it if you don't mind."

"All right, ma'am. It's your responsibility."

We chose a window table and she soon brought our meals. The pie was scrumptious with gluten-free pastry and came with a salad and olive oil and lemon juice dressing on the side. She was a very fine chef.

Overcoming a Sweet Tooth

Back in 2010, soon after starting to read about cancer, I'd realized that for many years I'd been consuming way too much sugar – not sugars hidden in processed foods because I hardly ate any processed food – but proudly conspicuous sugar that I chose for pleasing my sweet tooth.

- Hot fudge sundaes with two scoops, extra syrup and whipped cream;
- Cream puffs;
- Tiramisu;
- Chocolate eclairs;
- Chocolate bars with nuts and boxes of chocolates;
- Chocolate cheesecake;
- Pecan and pumpkin pies with piles of whipped cream.

I'd had one or two of these treats every week, all with coffee containing flavored creamer. Now as I read about cancer, it sank into my reluctant mind that I would have to stop all this, that my sweet tooth was gigantic and would have to be shrunk down to a safe size.

I was lucky in that my Dad had set me an example. Growing up, I had marveled at his sugarless cups of tea and preference for dark chocolate over milk chocolate.

"How can you drink it like that, Dad? It tastes awful!"

"Well, Jenny Wren, I had a sweet tooth once but the Great Depression came and things were scarce and we had little money. So one day I decided to give up sugar. And since that day, I haven't put sugar in tea or coffee, ever."

"Just in one day you stopped wanting sugar?"

"No, it took one day to stop using it and a few months to stop wanting it. Your milk chocolate tastes bad to me now."

He had retrained his taste buds and now I had to do the same. Since May, 2012, I've used no sugar in anything though I do buy 85% dark chocolate sometimes and I do use xylitol sometimes. (**Caveat**: one should only use xylitol obtained from the inner bark of birch trees, much as maple syrup is obtained from maple trees. Avoid the xylitol made from GMO corn.)

Coconut aminos now taste both tart and sweet to me. I even taste a little sweetness in non-pie pumpkin, which I detested since childhood for its bitter taste. And a lot of sweetness in fried onions. So I've found that using less sweetness teaches the palate to notice it more and be happy with less. There are some other good sweeteners besides stevia and xylitol:

- Erythritol, like xylitol, is a sugar alcohol. Neither is alcohol or sugar; they are organic compounds derived from sugars. Other examples you might notice on processed food labels are mannitol and sorbitol. They don't cause tooth decay, affect insulin production or feed cancer.

- Lakanto is made from Erythritol and monk fruit grown in the Himalayas. Monk fruit contains no fructose; instead it is sweetened by compounds called mogrosides. Lakanto comes in two forms: white looking like ordinary sugar and golden brown looking like raw sugar. I believe both taste like sugar and are water-soluble.

Items to Delete From an Anti-Cancer Diet

In all the discussion and controversy about what to eat and not eat against cancer, there is really quite a bit of agreement. The rule against eating sugar is unanimous because glucose, the digested form of sugar and all carbohydrates, is what feeds cancer cells. Since sugar comes in many disguises, here are four aspects of "no sugar" :

1. **No processed foods**. Virtually all of them are loaded with high fructose corn syrup (HFCS) that's 20% sweeter than natural sugar. Forget those center aisles in supermarkets – all those boxes, bottles and packets contain not only HFCS

but also chemicals (listed on their packaging or not) that have no business being in the human body. Their purpose is to benefit the food companies, e.g. fake colors, flavors and aromas that are cheaper and preservatives for longer shelf life to allow storage and exporting. Everyone knows that color, flavor and aroma are part of a good meal but processing removes much of those original qualities and the fake ones, laboratory chemicals, tend to be harmful to the body – slow toxins.

2. **No Soda Drinks**. This is an extension of "no processed foods" since soda drinks are just processed liquids loaded with sugar. Diet sodas are equally harmful as they contain Aspartame (sold as Equal and NutraSweet). Controversy swirls around Aspartame, with governments and corporations ("The Establishment") defending it and medical professionals explaining its many negative side effects. It's all easily found online. As a cancer patient I avoid it, using Xylitol, made from inner birch bark, as my sweetener; if one's health is in disarray, why eat possible poisons? Many people use stevia, derived from a plant.

3. **No Gluten**. Popular grains contain gluten, as most people know by now (wheat, oats, rye and barley); and gluten becomes glucose when we eat it. So even if you do not test as allergic to gluten, it's best to avoid it if you have cancer. There are gluten-free grains such as rice, quinoa and amaranth that we can eat in moderation and we can buy gluten-free pasta, cereals and breads. Keep grains as a minor part of your diet though, as, gluten or not, they all digest down to glucose.

4. **No alcohol.** Alcoholic drinks quickly become glucose after ingestion. The exception made here by some nutritionists is French red wine. It contains Resveratrol from red grapes and non-French red wines go through processing that destroys it. It's mostly in the seeds and skin and the French wine makers crush the grapes without removing seeds and skin. Resveratrol is an antioxidant that reduces inflammation and can cross the blood-brain barrier. Research studies have shown it to reduce the spread of cancer, lower blood pressure, and improve

heart health, among other benefits.* But aside from French red wine, we cancer patients should avoid alcohol. Another reason for that besides the glucose is that alcoholic drinks are acid-forming in the body. See "Little to no Coffee" below.

No Dairy Products. By the time we reach about five years of age, we have no more lactase, the enzyme for digesting cow's milk and its forms such as cheese and butter. This enzyme lack creates a sensitivity to dairy products as opposed to an allergy. It's an inability to digest them rather than a quick and visible reaction against them.

o   Yogurt can be an exception at times to "no dairy products" since it contains probiotics, but most commercial yogurt is loaded with sugar and has been pasteurized, which kills the bacteria we want. Coconut yogurt and kefir from health food stores are excellent alternatives.

o   There are two dairy ingredients that can cause allergic reactions: Lactose (milk sugar) and Casein (a milk protein). But even if you are not allergic to these items, avoid dairy products.

o   Another reason is that they are acid-forming in the body like coffee.

Little to no Coffee is also wise. The caffeine constricts blood vessels but a cancer patient needs them to be as open as possible so the blood can bring plenty of oxygen to all cells. Body cells become cancerous when oxygen is insufficient. Coffee is also acid-forming and cancer loves to be in acidic surroundings. A good anti-cancer diet needs to be more alkaline than acidic. See chapter 10 for more on that. (When coffee enters the body rectally, as in coffee enemas, it has entirely different effects. Please see p. 62-63 for more on this.)

---

* In more recent cancer research, a compound group called Salvestrols has been found. It is similar to Resveratrol but more powerful and supplements are available. It is processed in the body by our enzyme called CYP1B1 (SipOneBeOne) and the result is a metabolite that causes cancer cell death (apoptosis). See *Salvestrols: Nature's Defence Against Cancer*, listed on p 210. It's available on Amazon, as is a book on Salvestrol cancer case histories by the same author.

Well, that's surely enough prohibitions for the most Spartan among us!

Items to Include in an Anti-Cancer Diet

1. **Fresh Salads**. These should be a daily staple, large and full of colorful variety. Try to use only vegetables that are in season. When plants are forced out of season, they consist mostly of water and fiber, which are of course necessary in any good diet, but the plant's natural nutrition is largely absent. Shopping for organic vegetables at a Farmers Market is the simplest way to always have highly nutritious veggies. You can make it a fun social event too as there are usually tables and benches where you can sit with friends to sip your (infrequent) coffee and enjoy any of a large variety of meals provided. The only **Caveat** would be that the meals and coffee may not be organic. But some Farmers Markets are 100% organic.

   o Salad Dressings: Best to make your own. There are many for sale but they would all contain preservatives, probably at least one form of sugar, and maybe fake colors etc. Olive and coconut oil are excellent (though coconut oil will harden if you refrigerate it). I use these oils along with assorted other things such as lemon or lime juice, Bragg's Aminos, tahini and coconut milk or water for the right consistency.

2. **Green Juice and Smoothies**. Organic vegetable juice is one of the most beneficial things you can do for yourself. Make it mostly green though you can include a green apple or a few carrots or beets to taste; also a garlic clove or two and a squeeze of lemon or lime juice at the end.

   Juicing has become mainstream these days so perhaps you already have your own recipes. The idea is to ingest as many fresh, organic vegetables as possible to boost the blood with chlorophyll and oxygen. Smoothies can be entire meals and it's easy to find ideas and recipes online. A little caveat would be:

   o Beware of making them too sweet. Many smoothies offered by cafes and restaurants use a lot of fruit and the sweetest vegetables to make them more appealing to a public trained to like sugar.

3. **The Budwig Blend**. This is a mix of cottage cheese and flaxseed oil (CCFO) devised by Dr. Johanna Budwig about 70 years ago. She was a prominent research chemist in Germany, focusing largely on the structure of oils, and she discovered how important essential fatty acids are for good health. She discovered omega 3 and 6 fatty acids. See pp. 87-91 for more on and pp. 24-25 for more on Dr. Budwig.

If we lived in a kind and sensible world, CCFO would be given to every cancer patient the day they were diagnosed along with teaching on how to prepare it. It causes cancer cells to die and helps healthy cells to not become cancerous. Mix quark or low-fat cottage cheese (preferably with no preservatives) with fresh flaxseed oil in a two-to-one ratio. Anyone can benefit from this blend in any amount.

o   Use a hand-held mixer, not a standard blender.

The sulphur in the CC makes the FO water-soluble so it mixes into the CC and disappears from sight. This takes less than a minute. Once this chemical change happens, you can add fruit or cacao powder, nuts, seeds, honey, chopped onion, broccoli, or anything you like and the oil will not reappear. Since the oil is part of the CC, it is able to easily enter body cells for good nutrition and cancer cells for apoptosis (cell suicide).

o   If you have a food sensitivity to dairy products, not to worry. The CC loses its dairy properties and isn't CC any more, chemically. I have such a sensitivity but have no trouble with CCFO.

Some people find it tricky to blend. I find that this routine works:

o   Six rounded tablespoons CC with three tablespoons of oil. Mix a minute or so till oil is gone or mostly gone. Leave sitting for five minutes or so (covered). Mix again for about 20 seconds. If you still see oil, add a small amount of CC and mix briefly. This is a half dose (with vegetables or sometimes a little fruit). I fall asleep if I eat a full dose but if you prefer a full dose, just double it. The full CC amount in cups is two-thirds to three-quarters of a cup.

Caveat: Never buy FO off a store shelf, only from a refrigerator and only in a dark glass bottle. FO is fragile. It has a very low "smoking point" – the temperature at which it goes rancid. Air, light, and heat will all turn it rancid. The minute you've used it, cap it and replace it in the fridge.

For more on Dr. Budwig and her complete cancer diet, see the free download *Budwig Cancer Guide.pdf*, listed in *Print and PDF Resources.*

Eat 100% organic if you possibly can. Non-organic vegetables are sprayed many times as they grow; we can't wash off pesticides that have been incorporated into their growth. Anything genetically modified has built-in pesticides. This saves factory farms some money but it's a sure route to a leaky gut for us because those pesticides kill our gut-protective bacteria. I usually encounter a knee-jerk reaction against eating organic: "Oh, it's too expensive!" "Oh, I can't afford it!" However, a bit of thought will get anyone past that:

- Think of No Processed Food, things we usually buy from the center aisles of a supermarket and how much they cost. You can put that money towards organic foods and be far the better for it.

- The Budwig Blend is a full meal, especially with fruit or other add-ons, so there's more savings, of cooking time as well as money.

- Think further of how often you typically dine out. More savings because very few restaurants serve organic meals.

- Maybe you like a few drinks at a pub on weekends. Depending on your habits, this might be more savings.

How highly do you rate your health? Priorities can probably be changed. If you examine your usual budget you will surely find a few things you could do without for the sake of cancer recovery.

Other Food Items

The above discussion does not mention meats, fish, eggs or grains. There is controversy over these items. Cancer thrives in acidic surroundings so animal proteins are left out of some cancer diets because of having a highly acidic effect on the body's pH levels. Grains become glucose when digested, aside from whether they contain gluten or not, so some diets leave them out. They also have an acidic effect. You might be able to include all these items in moderation. Personally, I leave them out and just sometimes have some roast potato pieces from the local organic grocery store or some cassava root crackers with tahini and Bragg's Aminos. (Continued on p. 91)

Understanding Oils

If we habitually include the wrong oils and fats in our diet, we are jeopardizing our health in many ways. To better understand which oils are unhealthy and why, the first thing to do is dismiss everything we've heard and seen in the standard media. The second thing to do is get a clear understanding of the oil vocabulary. Words are thrown around every day without any definition of terms, and that causes us to repeat mantras like "Avoid saturated fats" without knowing what they mean.

I'm no chemist so I've had to study this subject and figure out which oils are truly safe to eat, which ones are safe to cook with (can tolerate heat), and which ones will go rancid too easily for safety, given that our health is already long-damaged if we have cancer.

Fats vs Oils

In the context of fats and oils, you may have heard the term *lipid*. It's a general term for both fats and oils. Fats and oils are very similar in composition (see below) but in general, fats originate in animals and oils originate in plants. A further distinction is that:

o   A fat is solid at room temperature and is more saturated (see below for explanation of "saturated");

o   An oil is liquid at room temperature and is less saturated.

However, this is relative because all oils will become solid at low enough temperatures and all fats will melt at high enough temperatures. The term "room temperature" is vague. Unless you have central heating and air conditioning, room temperature can be anything from freezing to sweltering, depending on many factors. But the term is standard in discussions of fats and oils so we have to interpret it as meaning "a comfortable temperature for daily living". Some discussions use the term "body temperature".

Fatty Acids and Triglycerides

The most important, frequent, and basic fats in the body are triglycerides. They make up our body fat. A triglyceride molecule (basic component consisting of an arrangement of atoms) consists of three fatty acids and a glycerol (also called glycerin).

o   Glycerol (or glycerin) is a viscous liquid lacking any color or odor.

Fatty acids fall into three groups:

1) Long chain fatty acids (LCFA)

2) Medium chain fatty acids (MCFA); and

3) Short chain fatty acids (SCFA).

Some are "essential fatty acids" without which our health would deteriorate to the point of death. So, as with "essential amino acids", the components of proteins, we need to include them in our diet.

Saturation

When a fat is "saturated", what is it saturated with? Hydrogen.

o   When it has as many hydrogen atoms as it has receptors for, it is saturated;

o   When it is missing just one hydrogen atom, it is mono-unsaturated;

o   When it is missing several or many hydrogen atoms, it is polyunsaturated.

Saturated fat is solid at "room temperature". Examples are butter and lard. Lard is pig fat that has been melted and strained ("rendered and clarified") to make it suitable for cooking. It was used a lot many years ago, in pastry and puddings and spread thickly on bread with a generous sprinkle of salt. Those were the days (my growing-up days in Australia and England) of home-grown vegetables and home-cooked meals, along with few overweight people and low incidence of cancer and diabetes. There is also suet – fat from around animal kidneys. It has a high smoking point, making it good for frying.

Hydrogenation

Lipids can be put through a chemical process to make them accept more hydrogen atoms than Nature designed them for and this is called hydrogenation. It makes the fatty acids solid at room temperature. Hydrogenated peanut butter is a solid mass but natural peanut butter has the oil separate at the top of the jar. Being an oil, it is liquid at room temperature. You then have to mix it in to get smooth spreadable peanut butter. (This bit of work is well worth it for your long-term health.)

Trans Fats

When a saturated fat is partially hydrogenated, it is called a trans fat. These fats are always harmful – they clog up our arteries and make heart disease more likely. They stop the arteries from making a substance called prostacyclin and the lack of prostacyclin promotes blood clots. These are dangerous because traveling in the blood, they can become lodged in the brain, causing a stroke, or in the heart, causing cardiac arrest.

Food companies are not required to include trans fats in the list of ingredients if it is a small amount per serving. So many processed foods have hidden trans fats. The best way to avoid trans fats is to avoid all processed foods.

Canola Oil

The canola oil that I used so freely and happily in Canada and before that in Denver was devised in the 1970s from rapeseed oil and since "rapeseed" doesn't sound very enticing, it was given a new name, with the "can" part from "Canada" and the "ola" indicating oil, cf. Mazola (corn or maize oil). There is no canola plant. Plants and crops given that name can be any of the several thousand members of the Brassicaceae family (also called Cruciferous) that includes broccoli, cabbage, cauliflower, alyssum and wallflowers.

For years canola oil was used in lipstick, biofuels, lubricants, insecticides and soap. Then in 1995 a genetically modified version was devised that we see in supermarkets. It has been put through procedures of bleaching, refining and degumming which all involve high temperatures or chemicals not suitable in foods. The high temperatures make the omega 3 fatty acid molecules go rancid and smell bad. So it's put through a deodorization procedure that converts the omega 3 to trans fat. As far as I know, no bottle of canola oil includes "trans fats on its ingredients list.

Polyunsaturated Fats

These are oils that could accept more than one more hydrogen atom. There are two kinds:

o   Those high in Omega 3 fatty acids; and

o   Those high in Omega 6 fatty acids.

We need both. Typically, people these days are over-supplied with Omega 6 and under-supplied with Omega 3. Like every imbalance in the body, this opens a person to health deterioration. Fish oil supplements are the most common way of correcting the imbalance as they are high in Omega 3. An example of an oil high in Omega 6 would be corn oil.

In their natural state, all oils are a mix of saturated, mono-unsaturated, and poly-unsaturated molecules. Their components, the fatty acids, are any of those three types of oil molecules. But usually one type predominates so that oil is talked of as being just that predominant type.

Rancidity

Heat, light and oxygen all cause rancidity. Every oil has a smoking point, where heat will start changing its chemistry, making it harmful to ingest. You can see it giving off smoke from the frying pan. Two oils that are particularly prone to rancidity are:

o   Canola oil where the chemical breakdown of rancidity starts happening before it reaches its smoking point.

o   Flaxseed oil (also called linseed oil), which has an extremely low "smoking point" such that no stove heat is necessary – "room temperature" will cause it to break down. You may have heard or read that flaxseed oil is highly healthful, and it is, but it's also fragile, which is why it's sold in a dark glass bottle, perhaps also in a box, and requires refrigeration. Never buy it off a store shelf. There's no telling whether it sat out in the sun waiting to be loaded on or off a truck. We can't tell if it's rancid by sniffing it as its rancidity generates no smell.

Restaurants re-use the same oil for fried dishes. Whatever oil they use, once it has been heated for making French Fries, for example, its smoking point is lower. It is now partially damaged chemically and when it's used again, it gets damaged at lower temperatures – and so on, until it's finally discarded. Somewhere in that sequence – maybe right at the start, depending on what oil it is and how high it gets heated -- it becomes rancid, assuming it started out fresh. Walking past some cafes or restaurants, you can smell the rancidity.

Rancidity involves creation of free radicals that do much damage in the body, speeding up our aging. Oxygen in the air mixes with the oil's molecules and another term for this is oxidation. The more an oil is processed, the more likely it is to become rancid because the fresh oil's antioxidants are destroyed. One cannot always tell by sniffing or tasting since processing will include deodorization.

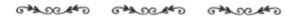

The Many Advantages of Coconut Oil

For many years in America and perhaps elsewhere, coconut oil has been misrepresented by standard media outlets and by many websites. Truth is often thrown out when it comes to marketing products and there have been some lies told many times about coconut oil. The people engaged in this deception hid or ignored the fact that there are several kinds of saturated fat and coconut oil is not the type that raises cholesterol.

- Coconut oil is a saturated fat that does **not** raise your cholesterol.

(By the way, cholesterol is made and needed in the body to keep blood vessels limber and flexible; this has been another marketing or media hype, that cholesterol is harmful.) Coconut oil is entirely health-promoting with no undesirable side effects. It is 90% Medium Chain Fatty Acids (MCFAs) which makes it a very different food than the Long Chain Fatty Acid oils. When we ingest MCFAs, they do not get deposited in our fat cells. They go to the liver which converts them into energy. An advantage flowing from this fact is that if we substitute coconut oil for other oils in our diet, we will gradually lose weight (assuming we are not over-eating).

Other coconut oil advantages are:

- It tolerates pretty high heat so it makes a good cooking oil. Just don't heat it so much that it smokes (toss it out if that happens).

- It is anti-bacterial, anti-viral and anti-fungal. It functions in these ways both inside the body and on the skin thereby preventing or alleviating hundreds of health problems and a short list of examples would be throat infections, food poisoning, skin eruptions, influenza and herpes.

- It is high in Omega 3 fatty acids which are deficient in most people. They should be balanced 1:1 with Omega 6 fatty acids.

- It makes an excellent skin emollient. Forget those expensive skin lotions and creams!

- It causes no harm to the cardiovascular system.

- It is a mild sunscreen, blocking about 20% of the sun's UV rays.

- It is an antioxidant, combatting free radicals and helping to prevent premature aging.

Coconuts are made into many different products besides oil. We can buy coconut milk, water, cream, aminos (a sauce like tamari), syrup, flour, "crunch" (for sprinkling on porridge or yogurt, for example), flakes, and paste, all with different uses in food preparation. We can also buy coconut soap, shampoo, and conditioner; and scrubbers for the shower or bath that are made from the fibrous outer covering of older coconuts.

Personally, I was introduced to coconuts in Costa Rica. Greg and I were walking along the waterfront in Puerto Viejo, admiring the bamboo furniture and hand-made clothing and jewelry (at least I was), and we came to a man with a barrow of coconuts who said,

"You want a delicious cool drink?"

We did, so he seized his small machete with one hand and a coconut with the other and with five well-placed strikes he made a neat hexagonal opening in the top of the coconut (a young coconut without the fibrous covering). He placed a straw in the opening and made another for Greg. We gave him some colones (Costa Rica currency) and big smiles and continued our sunny stroll. That (fresh!) coconut water was very thirst-quenching and satisfying and we became repeat customers.

Later, in Thailand, I got a kitchen machete and made such drinks often. Coconut water is brimming with vitamins, minerals, enzymes, electrolytes, amino acids, and phytonutrients. Once the coconut is opened and we've drunk the fresh water, we can spoon out all the meat and with clean water in a blender, make coconut milk.

As the saying goes, We are What we Eat. And as the more accurate saying goes, We are What We Digest. What we absorb through our digestive system plays a huge role in our health and strength; and what we **don't** absorb plays an equally huge role through its absence.

It's not really hard to change one's diet. Once we acknowledge that our habitual diet has been less than optimum for good health, it's enjoyable to explore new foods, try new recipes, and buy new kitchen appliances and see what they can do. If you are feeding a family, they will all benefit from the changes and your children will grow up wiser and healthier.

What to do Next?

By December 2012, I had been receiving treatments at the Arizona clinic for eight months, way longer than most people. For the first four months, I relied on the raw vegan meals supplied by the Clinic kitchen and accepted whatever treatments Dr. Lodi ordered.

After four months, I was a lot stronger and healthier and a great deal of my money was gone. I asked Dr. Benson,[*] one of the naturopaths and the staff person I talked with about my health every Friday, if I could reduce the frequency of treatments and number of supplements. He was a natural born healer and a very kind and attentive person. We had good rapport. So on this Friday after the four months, we went through all my supplements and treatments and reduced their number for a new maintenance protocol. I became a part-time patient, feeling enormously better than when Dmitri had brought me to the clinic, unable to walk or stay awake very long.

Starting in the fifth month, I prepared my own raw vegan food in my apartment. The Clinic kitchen staff lent me their dehydrator over some weekends and I shared it with Margaret of colonics fame. From recipes in the Oasis "cookbook", we made flat bread, crackers and wraps from nuts and seeds and kept them in the freezer for a month's supply or so. I was still pushing the walker to and from Oasis and still received IV treatments

---

[*] Not his real name.

like chelation, Vitamin C, ALA, and IPT. I also still bought green juice from Oasis but I used my VitaMix to make soups, pates, and sauces. I also made cream cheese from cashews and Rejuvelac (fermented water made from rye berries) and "parmesan" cheese from brazil nuts and brewer's yeast.

When Dr. Lodi was absent from the clinic, he was often in Bangkok, apparently networking there, getting to know medical people. One day he appeared in the doorway of one of the treatment rooms, a place where he could see patients in two of the treatment rooms and they could see and hear him. He sometimes gave us a motivating pep talk from that doorway.

On this day, he announced that he had made arrangements in Bangkok for any of us to have stem cell treatments. Someone would meet us at the Bangkok airport and drive us to the facility offering the treatments, then drive us to a hotel or back to the airport. Food would be provided.

This idea caught my interest immediately. I had read that stem cells were effective in treating leukemia and I felt that my time at Oasis was finished. The intensive IV treatments along with the raw vegan diet and other treatments such as infrared saunas, acupuncture, colonics, and lymphatic drainage had made my health vastly better so that I felt energetic and optimistic. But according to the CBCs (Complete Blood Count), I still had leukemia. I also still had the partial hearing loss and the balance problem and needed the walker, and I'd sold my house in Denver. So what should I do next?

I made the decision quickly and told Dr. Lodi I was ready to go whenever the stem cell people were ready for me. There was some delay but on January 12 2013, I flew to Thailand. My plan was to stay there for a few months and possibly have several stem cell treatments, hoping to then be cancer free. Dr. Lodi was now employed part-time at a Thai spa outside of Chiang Mai, Thailand's second largest city. It was called Tao Garden and he was the clinic doctor there as well as still directing Oasis in Arizona. He would be traveling back and forth. He had arranged accommodation for me near Tao Garden and although he wouldn't be there when I arrived, he would arrive soon after.

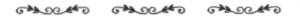

Memorandum

✓ Whether your diet is raw vegan or not, you will be headed for improved health if you eat organic.

✓ With persistence and patience you can overcome a sweet tooth and avoid sugar that would otherwise feed your cancer.

✓ Items to exclude from an effective anti-cancer diet are processed foods and drinks; gluten; alcohol; and dairy products.

✓ Items to include in such a diet are: fresh salads; green juice and smoothies; the Budwig Blend; and 100% organic food if you possibly can.

✓ Shun trans fats but include coconut oil in your diet.

✓

✓

✓

Chapter 6: Stem Cell Treatments in Thailand

My plane landed in Bangkok where I changed airline and flew north to Chiang Mai. It was now about midnight. When I walked out from the security and customs areas, there was a one-man welcoming crowd, a smiling man holding a sign with my name on it. Dr. Lodi had arranged for him to drive me to my new home.

"Jen-ee-FER?"

"Yes." Despite my fatigue, I felt a laugh gurgling in me at the way he said my name – not how I usually reacted when called Jennifer. In my world thus far, nobody called me "Jennifer" unless they were mad at me. But this was something in another world. I started adapting at that moment: he's not upset with me, my plane wasn't late, he speaks Thai.

In fact, he was my new landlord and I'll call him Anurak. In warm, humid darkness, we drove for about 45 minutes through Chiang Mai and out northwards. I couldn't see much of the surroundings and my fatigue was making me nod off a bit but Anurak was good-humored and didn't seem to mind. With his English limited and my Thai non-existent, we sat in comfortable silence. We drove off the main road on to a winding side road and through a village, then on to a smaller side road with no paving. We passed an area more brightly lit with a gateway and a guard on duty.

"Tao Garden," said Anurak, pointing. "You walk there."

A few yards further, left turn into a stony dirt pathway barely wide enough for a car, and there was my bungalow. Anurak carried my two suitcases and unlocked the door and I stumbled in, ready for bed. Anurak gave me the door key and left. He lived at the other end of the pathway, as I learned later, past a series of bungalows that he owned and rented out. Dr. Lodi had arranged for me to rent the one closest to Tao Garden. They were all part of the village called Doi Saket that surrounded Tao Garden. My bungalow had two rooms and a bathroom. No kitchen. Two fans but no air conditioner. A single bed. I quickly got ready to use it, finding hot water in the bathroom of the kind that heats up as you use it – hot water on demand so no tank. I'd had no dinner but the bungalow's little fridge, the height of my chest, was empty.

When I woke in the morning, the birds were vigorous and noisy. "You alright? You alright?" "Surreal! Surreal!" "It's Macau twit" "No, twit, it's Cacao!" "Cheap, cheap, cheap." Sunbeams filled the little bedroom and looking out the window, I noticed a lake or pond across the dirt road. There were lots of trees shading the bungalow and lake and other bungalows across the lake. Dogs were barking and to my right, a baby was crying. There was no clock but I had my trusty iPhone and it told me that breakfast was now being served in the Tao Garden dining room.

I got dressed, putting on a hat to cover my bald head, and pushed my walker out the door, down the step, and out onto the dirt road. It was bumpy and I weaved carefully back and forth avoiding rocks and potholes that could have stopped the walker abruptly and had me sprawled across it. Out the driveway to the main village road and turn right. A big rice field was now on my left with a couple of people, wearing tall pointed hats, bending over to do something with the young plants. I crossed five little streams or canals that ran to the rice field. The walk was short to that gate we had passed last night – only about five minutes.

I smiled at the guard and entered the Tao Garden property. Flowers were everywhere. Gardeners were already at work watering and trimming, big hats shading their faces. There was a river to my left, flowing vigorously, and I later learned that it was controlled by a nearby dam and watered all the neighboring rice fields. There were rose bushes, bougainvillea, hibiscus, and as I breathed deeply of the clean air, I noticed gardenias, my favorite scent. There were also many plants I didn't recognize and scores of fantastic orchids. The path was paved in octagonal red bricks and branched off to the left several times on bridges over the river.

Soon I came to an archway and bridge on my right among ancient-looking potted bonsai trees, hanging baskets of orchids, big tubs of flowers, and two big birdbaths with water lilies. I saw that the bridge led to a dining room with no walls and I could see people at a buffet and carrying trays and clustered at many tables. Along the bridge were two big painted urns and more flowers.

My first Thai breakfast was fried Morning Glory (there were no raw greens so I compromised by at least having cooked ones), and oatmeal with black sesame seeds and hot soy milk. I put these items on a tray on the walker seat and found a vacant chair at one of the crowded round tables. I added some brown sugar (not good for cancer) to the oatmeal and my own sea salt and started munching. Everybody was talking at once and I heard German, French and English.

"You must have just arrived," said a woman on my right.

I nodded, swallowing oatmeal and returning her smile.

"I'm Elizabeth," she offered. She was about 40 with blond hair and plump pink cheeks. I could hear that she spoke German but her English was good.

"Jen." I said. "Got here late last night."

"Well, I suppose you weren't up for Chee Gong then!"

"Were you?" I said, wondering what it was.

"Oh no, I teach classes here." The woman on her right claimed her attention then and they switched to German. Soon they left but Elizabeth patted my shoulder and said, "See you at lunch time."

I was good and had no coffee; instead I tried the ginger tea.

Many people had left to begin their day now and I could see the surrounding structures better. There were 16 round tables each seating seven. The dining room was situated in a lake and all exits were bridges. I saw some people tossing morsels of bread into the lake, evidently feeding the fish. Leaving half the ginger tea, I pushed the walker over a different bridge than the one I had entered on and found it led to a Juice Bar, also with no walls except the back one behind the counter. There were some couches and easy chairs with small wicker tables and two young women behind the counter. The chunky woman was preparing coffees for the group on one of the couches who seemed to be speaking Russian.

I smiled at the slim woman and looked at the sign propped on the counter giving the ingredients of a "Sunshine Cheer". It looked similar to the Oasis green juice so I asked for one.

"Yeh. You sit down. We bring for you," said the slim woman, exuding competence and friendliness.

"Thanks," I said, feeling suddenly more at home. I counted out the right colorful money and placed it on the counter. Then I stationed the walker out of people's way and leaned back on the fat cushions of a wicker love seat. Already the day was warm and I noticed two big standing fans that would no doubt be used before long. I had brought a book under the walker seat and I put it on the wicker table, enjoying the many birds in the surrounding trees. A black and white bird was perched on the Juice Bar railing and filling the building like an opera soprano belting out her agonies. Maybe calling his partner, I thought, since he was alone and no bird was joining him. My mind drifted away to the crowd of colorful lorikeets I used to feed on my Dad's balcony railing in Sydney. They loved pieces of bread soaked in honey water.

"Here your green joo."

The slim woman placed a tall glass full of green on the glass tabletop. I smiled and so did she, and immediately we had a rapport. It lasted my entire time at Tao Garden. I'll call her Kim. Taking a juice break became almost a daily little event and after a few weeks, I knew to say "Kob kun kaaa" – thank you (from a female – from a male it would have been "Kob Kun Ka" said more percussively and without the gracious trail upwards). It turned out that Kim took in people's laundry and soon I was bringing her a plastic bag each week of jumbled clothes and the next day picking them up neatly folded with an itemized note taped on the bag stating the amount owed.

On this first day though, I sat for a while sipping the juice and looking at the people coming and going. Some ordered coffee, made in the Thai style with very strong black coffee first, topped with hot milk. Thailand grows most of the coffee served in cafes and restaurants, though rice is the biggest crop, largely exported. As I was finishing the juice and wondering whether to walk around Tao Garden some more, stay put and read my book, *The Biology of Belief* by Bruce Lipton (about Epigenetics), or go back to the bungalow and unpack, a young nurse approached me, wearing white cap, white shoes and white stockings to complete her white uniform. I remembered my own days as a nurse, when I had worn a similar cap and uniform with my name tag pinned in front. I'm glad that American nurses wear colored scrubs these days and casual shoes good for the feet and no cap.

"You are Jen-ee-FER?"

"Yes."

"The doctor wait for you."

I squinted up at her, the bright light shining on her long black hair and in my eyes. She was like a perfectly designed nurse-doll, beautiful to look at, compact and dainty. By comparison I felt oversized.

"Dr. Lodi is still in America," I said.

"Dr. Palo* wait for you."

OK. So the clinic had several doctors. It was nice that this doctor knew I'd arrived. I got up, put my book under the walker seat, and maneuvered myself out of the juice bar. The clinic entrance was just a few yards away on the opposite side of the pathway and the nurse held the door open for me. Though I saw umpteen pairs of shoes carelessly kicked off outside this door, I kept my sandals on because to take them off, I needed to sit down. Inside the door there was a bench with a boxful of slippers to wear inside the clinic. I removed my sandals, put on a pair of beige scuffs from the box, and looked around. The nurse was waiting for me so I followed her across the large entrance area, with two groups of coffee table and wicker chairs, comfortably cushioned, past the reception counter where several young women were bustling and phoning, and to a partially open door on the left side of a corridor. The nurse turned back to the counter and I knocked on the door, as I couldn't see anyone in there yet.

"Yes, come in," came a rich-sounding baritone.

I pushed the walker through and met the gaze of a muscular young black man seated at the desk. He had looked away from his computer monitor to see who was entering and our eyes remained locked for a few moments. I felt suddenly and completely at home and glad I was there and at the same time, suddenly exposed. His perceptive gaze saw instantly through my surface to me, myself.

He silently said hello to me on a spirit level and I returned the hello. Then we both remembered our manners and I smiled and he got up to greet me.

"Welcome to Tao Garden, Jennifer."

He pulled one of the chairs away from my side of his desk and gestured that I should sit.

"Thanks," I said, in something of a daze.

---

* Not his real name

"How was your trip? I believe you got in quite late last night?"

"Yes, um … midnight or so. Anurak picked me up. My landlord."

He seemed relaxed. His head was shaved and he had curly eyelashes and was wearing a short-sleeved green surgical shirt. My eyes kept going to his long elegant fingers, until I remembered my manners again and tried to recall what he had just said. His level gaze saw straight into me without actually invading my space – he wasn't throwing energy my way, just sizing me up.

"Do you work with Dr. Lodi?" I said.

"Yes, I fill in for him when he's away in Bangkok or America." I could hear no accent in his English; he sounded like any other (non-Southern) American, but his energy seemed different.

"So he's arranging stem cell treatments in Bangkok and also running this clinic?"

"He is the head doctor here, yes. He gets around." Dr. Palo grinned at my confusion. "He's starting a cancer clinic in Bangkok. He has some partners."

This information made sense and answered some questions I'd had.

"Are you a cancer doctor?" I asked.

"Yes, a cancer surgeon. My training and experience have all been in America. I lived there for about 20 years."

"Where are you from then?"

"Zambia."

I conjured up a map of Africa but Zambia wasn't on it. "Where's Zambia?"

"It used to be Northern Rhodesia, a British colony. Now it's an independent country." This information shed light on my puzzlement about his voice --- Zambia is an English-speaking African country, hence his speech had no accent other than American replacing his British-sounding speech. Same as me; my American voice (after 42 years living there) mostly replaced my Aussie one.

Dr. Palo watched the puzzle pieces slipping into place in my brain. When I looked up at him again, my heart was bubbly with laughter and there was no place I wanted to be other than in his company.

"Well, Dr. Palo, what should we do now?" I asked.

"If you don't mind, I'd like to get your vitals and order a CBC for you. We need to see what your white cells are doing."

This was familiar territory – chronic myeloid leukemia causes an elevated white count, elevated platelets, and reduced red cells. He took his stethoscope from the coat stand and listened to my heartbeat, put a digital thermometer in my mouth, and took my blood pressure. Then he went to the doorway and called over to the front desk,

"Ying, could you take a blood sample from Jennifer please?"

Ying was the nurse who had fetched me from the juice bar.

"I still have a port," I said, showing her the dangling end on my upper right chest. She first flushed the port with a saline solution, then inserted her syringe into it, thus giving me no pain from any needle stick, and withdrew several ccs of blood. Then she taped the end of the port to my chest.

"You like ginger tea?" she asked.

I said Yes, thinking I should learn to enjoy it, and she led me out to the main entry area, gesturing to one of the bamboo chairs. I gave Dr. Palo a smile and followed her with my walker. There were two ceramic urns on a side table and she filled a little cup from one of them and brought it to me on its little saucer.

"You relak," she said. "You here long a' you like." She walked along the corridor to a back room and disappeared.

I leaned back, sipped my ginger tea and watched the comings and goings in and out of the clinic. Someone else was in Dr. Palo's office now. A group of people were sitting across the room at another set of bamboo chairs, speaking German. Being an inveterate wordsmith, I liked listening to different languages and German was somewhat familiar to me. To my impaired hearing much of their conversing simply muddled with the Thai being spoken at the front desk but occasional words floated some meaning my way – they brought Schubert songs to mind.

Life at Tao Garden

Tao Garden is a beautiful place! Almost everywhere you look there is high-quality, whether it's landscaping, flooring, tea cups or lunch. Everything is designed to please. There were over 100 people visiting and most lived in the Tao Garden housing. Some, like me, lived in external housing. For $320/month rent I got electricity, bottled water and bathroom tissue; plus cleaning done weekly with fresh sheets and a towel. Anurak, my landlord, responded promptly to my phone call one day about a broken light and he brought a young man with him.

"He a good worker," he said with a grin. "Me, I no good." So he rode off on his bike and the young man expertly fixed the light.

The dining room offers a scrumptious, but mostly cooked, array of vegetable dishes, fish and chicken, soup, rice, desserts, and a big salad bar. The raw vegan diet was now history. There were always fresh fruit and fruit juice, and drinks such as ginger tea and alkalinized water. Sometimes I had no idea what vegetables or fruit I was eating, but they looked and tasted good.

Thailand is a Buddhist country but in Tao Garden there were people from many countries and backgrounds, coming for a week or two, for specific classes or retreats, meeting up with acquaintances they hadn't seen since their last visit – a sort of loosely-structured club. The whole place is run by a Thai Buddhist Master who took his meals in the same dining room as the rest of us, at a special table where his wife and two small daughters could sit with him, or special guests. Somewhere in my first week, he gave me a friendly welcome, patting my arm and inviting me to join his Qi Gong class early each morning.

There was a Dark Room coming up in my second month there. At lunch one day people at my table were talking about it.

"Are you here for the Dark Room?" asked Howie*, a very tall German man who had spent much of his life in Phuket, the south part of Thailand that has many beautiful beaches. He had owned a restaurant there. He was sitting next to me at our round table.

---

* Not his real name

"No, Howie. I don't know about it." I said.

I did know which building was designated for it – one of the row of nice townhouses on the far side of Tao Garden's grounds. People could buy or rent these and they were all occupied, to my knowledge. Tao Garden staff had asked some people to move for the duration so one entire townhouse could be used for the Dark Room.

"Oh! Well, you must try it, Jen. It's starting on Sunday. Most of these new people are here for it."

"So what happens?"

"You have a room," he said. "All to yourself. Windows are blocked, you can't turn on the light, you stay in your room every day."

"What about meals? Does someone slide cheese and ham under the door?"

He laughed. "Oh, you can leave once a day for dinner but you mustn't talk. Nobody talks. Breakfast and lunch you get, somebody brings you a tray. And you have plenty of drinking water.

Part of me was marveling that so many people bought plane tickets and flew thousands of miles to sit alone in a dark room. But I knew the purpose.

"So you practice meditation," I said.

"Yes. With so much quiet and darkness and so much time on your hands, you must turn inwards."

"I'll bet some people have trouble with it," I commented, thinking of some of my own agonizing "growth periods", as they were called in California, when my energy work had stirred up some layer of old pain or anger and I was in the throes of letting it go. Sometimes that was done in a few moments but other times it took days or weeks and I'd needed help, a staff person to look at my energy and help me disengage from the old stuff.

Heinz grinned at me sideways a little. "You get through it," he said. Yes, I thought, he's had trouble with it himself. But here he was, back for more.

At Tao Garden, I was actually not very interested in the class offerings. My several years in California of spiritual training when I was in my 30s had been very intensive and pivotal in my life. They had transformed me, stripped off layer upon layer of energy accretions built up since my birth. I still used my energy tools daily and didn't want to get involved with an Asian approach to the same sort of thing.

During the week of the Dark Room, the dining room was quiet and in the absence of bustle, some local cats found me. They were the skinniest cats I'd ever seen, here in the midst of abundance. Naturally, I picked up good supplies of meat and fish from the buffet and dropped pieces under the table when a cat came by. I could see the little creatures trembling as they gulped the food down. I was told as I left the dining room one day that we weren't supposed to feed the cats. Well, I thought, someone has to since they're apparently not finding enough mice or birds to eat. So I continued to drop chunks for them, discreetly, and thankfully only one or two ever came by at the same time.

A Jolt in my Improving Health

Around the dining room were three little gazebos where you could have your meal alone or talking to someone privately. One day I took my tray to one of them and got started eating but before long, a strange feeling came over me. I started to shake and feel cold. I buttoned up my travel cardigan and sipped the hot ginger tea but I grew colder until I became alarmed. Got to get into bed, I thought, and I left the tray there, wheeling the walker over the bridge back to the dining room as fast as I could walk, then over the bridge to the main path, out the gate and back to the bungalow. I put the extra blanket on the bed and curled up fully dressed and covered to my chin. Thailand's weather had been rather cool when I arrived but was now warmer so why was I feeling so chilled? I could have gone to see Dr. Palo but instead I fell asleep and on waking late afternoon, things were normal again. No shakes and shivers. Over the next few nights, this happened twice more but sleep took care of it and in between, I felt entirely normal.

About a week later, it happened again more severely. I was in the Juice Bar reading and now Dr. Lodi was also at Tao Garden, so this time I went to his office in the clinic.

"D-d-doctor Lodi, I'm very c-c-cold and I d-d-don't know why."

He saw me shivering and had me lie on the patient guerney in his office with a blanket over me. He called a nurse in to take my vitals.

"M-m-more b-b-blankets p-p-please."

"Ying, go and find another blanket," he said, and took my blood pressure himself. Ying came back with another blanket but even under two, I was enormously cold and shaky.

"The clinic ha no more blanket," said Ying.

"M-more b-b-blankets!" I kept saying, raising it to a shout. Dr. Palo was there now, apparently finished with his other patient. Dr. Lodi felt my forehead and patted my shoulder. "We'll find more blankets," he said soothingly, in a voice I'd never heard him use before. I was only half-conscious of anything going on around me now but did notice that both doctors left the room. That prompted more calls of "More blankets please" and after a while, the doctors returned with a nurse who placed two more blankets over me.

"We had to search and we finally got these from the housing," said Dr. Lodi. He set me up with an IV pole, the tubing inserted into my port. Finally warm enough, I fell asleep. I woke to see Dr. Palo entering the room to check on me.

"How are you feeling, Jen?"

I considered a moment. "Much better," I said in some surprise. I had felt so awful so recently. In another hour or so I was able to get up and push my walker home to the bungalow. There were no more episodes of those chills nor a name for them, and I forgot to ask what was in the IV. I'd guess high-dose vitamin C for some kind of tropical fever. I continued to wait for the first stem cell treatment.

Dragged to the Gym

One day soon after this I was relaxing in the Juice Bar at one of the bamboo and glass tables with a cup of coffee and with my laptop sitting idle for a change. Normally I checked email and wrote to a few friends and read things about cancer. This day I was in my right brain world, half-listening to the mix of languages from across the room. It was German from one table and French from the other. Some German I knew from my first husband's Viennese family and from German music. French I used to know well enough to read novels and plays. I recalled those French books, printed on thick grainy paper with every other page continuous with the following one, so you had to use a letter opener (remember those?) to separate each pair of pages. In Australia I never met a French person to talk with so my seven years learning the language had all been academic. Yet, I mused, in Costa Rica, when I spoke what Spanish I could, what first came to mind were French words: *dejeuner, petite, garçon* …

The sun was glittering on the pond water and making the tub of red poppies brilliant and a voice said,

"Hello Jen. May I sit here?"

It was Dr. Palo and I came to and said, "Yes, you certainly can."

He had coffee too. If you have cancer, coffee is controversial. Some ban it because it's acidic and cancer cells love acidity. Also the caffeine constricts blood vessels, cutting down on the oxygen brought to body cells by the red blood cells. This creates a more favorable environment for body cells to turn cancerous like their neighbors. They copy their neighbors much the way some people do. Other cancer experts allow some coffee because it's sociable and pleasant and helps cancer patients relax and they argue that emotional benefits are as important as physical negatives. So although typically I had green juice rather than coffee, on this day I felt like being out of the box for a while.

"How are you feeling today?" asked Dr. Palo. It wasn't a platitude as with idle chatter; it was a doctor's question following up on that recent shivering episode.

"Pretty good today. Feeling restless though. You got a break between patients?"

"I do. I've had two cases of Dengue Fever this week. Had to take one of them to hospital yesterday. Why don't you go to the gym and work off your restlessness?"

"Oh no. I've never been in a gym. At least, not unless it was all cleared for dancing."

Dr. Palo leaned back in the bamboo chair and fixed his intense black eyes on me.

"I think it's time you got acquainted with gyms. They have a nice one here, just down that path." He waved towards the path running past the Juice Bar.

"Yeah." Silence. I'd seen it because it was next to the swimming pool. A pool is something I can relate to, if it doesn't have chlorine in it, an established carcinogen. This one was salt water. I'd been going there for a while, using one of their available swimsuits, since

I hadn't brought mine with me from Costa Rica via Arizona, and getting help from the young man who was usually working there when I arrived. There were three stone steps between the dressing room and pool and they inspired panic in me. No railing. I just couldn't step down them but Kiet usually noticed me hesitating there, as he moved reclining chairs around or collected floaties.

"Want bit of help?" he'd say, his wide grin flashing at me. He stood at my shoulder height or so. He'd offer a sturdy arm as a railing and I'd carefully step down three times.

"Big thank you!" I'd say, or "Kob kun kaaa", and he'd nod and continue working. I didn't dive in, being afraid I wouldn't know which way was Up once I got underwater. I'd noticed that I relied on visual cues for walking, not on any internal sense of up and down. So I climbed down the ladder in the shallow end and then, in one of my natural elements (others being dance floors, orchestra pits and choir risers), swam 12 or more lengths, increasing the number as I gradually got stronger. But a gym???

"Well?" Dr. Palo said, grinning at my reluctance. "Come on. I'll show you what to do. Finish your coffee and meet me there in ten minutes, OK?"

He returned his cup to the counter and strode back to the clinic, across the side path. Soon I sighed and returned my cup to the counter and closed my laptop.

"Can I leave this computer here?" I asked Kim. "Going to the gym."

"Yeh, I put it behind counter here."

I gave her a thumbs up and headed for the pool and gym area. One lovely thing along this part of the pathway was the two gardenia bushes. I could sniff that heady aroma well ahead of reaching the bushes. I pushed the walker to the covered area that gives access to dressing rooms on one side and the gym on the other and parked it outside the gym door.

Dr. Palo was already there, flat on the floor and lifting what looked like hugely heavy weights. I leaned on the attendant's desk and watched as he finished his sequence. He was clearly at home in a gym.

"Come over here and I'll show you the machines I think you could use."

Without the walker, I put a hand here and there on machines for balance and followed him to the big windows at one side.

"Step up here," he said. Each side of this equipment had a railing so I complied with ease and looked at the dial. He glanced at my hands on those rails and pressed the On button. Immediately I was jounced and jiggled in a crazy rapid fashion. I laughed and gripped those railings more firmly.

"What the heck is this for?"

"It stimulates the lymph and blood circulation. It's set to run for ten minutes. So just relax and there's a timer there you can check." He walked to another machine and continued his own routine.

I stood being jiggled and gazed at the bright flowers along the path outside the glass wall. There were some huge black bees visiting them. My heart weeps for our bees possibly disappearing from the planet. That's a cause for genuine concern, in my view. We'd all starve without the bees pollinating our plants but the pesticides are killing the bees. Mass farming methods are killing our soil and friendly insects as well as poisoning our air and food. The machine suddenly went still and my brain took a moment to come into the here and now.

Stepping down, I glanced around for Dr. Palo and there he was, approaching.

"How did you like that? Easy or what? Let's go to the other side and do another machine." As I started walking, reaching for the next equipment to steady myself, he said,

"Jen, walk from your hips."

I stopped, puzzled, and he walked away from me. "Take each step from the hip like this. Swing your leg forward."

I imitated him and realized I'd been mincing around with smaller steps than natural. I was afraid of falling. I hadn't fallen at all since the stroke took my balance but I still feared it. Not knowing where Up is I felt a fear of losing the visual cues so I walked carefully keeping an eye on them.

In regard to where Up is: after my time in Thailand, I went to Costa Rica with Dmitri — he flew from New York and we met up at Atlanta airport to finish the trip together. The goal was to retrieve as many as possible of my now-moldy belongings stored at my old cottage in Puerto Viejo. When that was done we had a free afternoon so we spent it at the Puerto Viejo beach. Dmitri had not been to a beach since I last took him in Sydney when he was four but after some initial caution, he ventured further out in the waves. I stayed in the shallows for fear of being knocked over.

But sure enough, a larger wave did knock me over. Underwater, I had no idea where Up was and just flailed around. But Dmitri had been keeping an eye on me so he got to me quickly and pulled me upright. I was pretty shaken up by that. As a teen on Sydney beaches each January, I'd been fearless and to catch the biggest waves would have been the furthest person out, were it not for my Dad's rule:

- Jenny Wren, never be the furthest out. We have life guards but that doesn't mean a hungry shark won't get you before the guards see it.

So I was always the second furthest out. In those days we used heavy rubber rafts called glides. They were rented at every beach for a shilling a day and were excellent for riding waves (on your belly, not standing up). Later, they were outlawed because they too often bonked people on the head as we rode them to shore. They were hard and heavy so maybe they caused head injuries sometimes though I'd never seen anything approaching that in the years I used them. I was in America when they were outlawed and was very disappointed to return ten years later and find people using styrofoam boogie boards. Not half as much fun.

Back to the Tao Garden gym. Dr. Palo had me use the stationary bike and the treadmill and I had to agree that I did need this sort of gym work. The balance problem had kept me too sedentary for a year by that time. Body movement is so important for a cancer patient. One has to promote blood and lymph flow (a) so dead cancer cells and other departing toxins get carried to the kidneys or liver for excretion; and (b) so oxygen gets carried to each body cell. Lymph flow connects to venous blood in waste disposal while arterial blood, fresh from the lungs, carries the oxygen. The whole system must keep moving for the body to stay healthy.

Shortly after this, Dr. Lodi left Tao Garden. He had been traveling back and forth from Bangkok but now he stopped reappearing. I was in Thailand for stem cell treatments and was only at Tao Garden because Dr. Lodi had been in charge of the clinic and had organized my stay there. After he left, Dr. Palo became my doctor and took over the job of running the clinic.

First Stem Cell Treatment

From Arizona, Dr. Lodi emailed me that the stem cell clinic was ready now and I should book a ticket for Bangkok next week. Someone would meet me at the airport and I'd be well looked after.

Tao Garden's front entrance has a big circular driveway in front of the Welcome Building where there's a lot of coming and going. There's a bus that leaves twice a day to take people into Chiang Mai and it can be booked for airport runs too. On this morning, the bus and I arrived at the Welcome building on the dot of 8:30 am. It took 45 minutes to get to the airport. I had requested a wheelchair with my ticket though I was bringing my walker, as the wheelchair pusher would know where the gate was and I could relax about possibly missing the plane. At the check-in counter I asked for a window seat.

"Solly Ma'am, have wheelchair. If wheelchair, no window. Aisle seat."

I pouted a bit. "But I want to see Thailand!" It was a sunny day with just a bit of haze.

She smiled slightly but was adamant. I suppose if you're in a wheelchair, they think you might be incontinent too and can't be trusted at a window seat. But when we took off, the two seats next to me were empty so I had a window seat anyway. It's such a short flight (one hour) that no sooner do you achieve cruising altitude than you start descending. Thailand is a very well-watered place with rivers and lakes of every size, along with canals and some man-made lakes, all for watering rice paddies. From the air, it looks about half cultivation and half housing. All green and pretty with smallish areas of ridged mountains.

I was met in Bangkok by two members of the clinic staff, a young nurse I'll call Mali who presented me with a bright yellow "lei" like in Hawaii, and a young man I'll call Chati who drove the taxi, which evidently functions as the company shuttle.

"Are you a vegetarian?" Mali asked me as we drove through the city. I said Yes (reluctantly – I still missed those eggs sunny side up with hash browns and cheese and bacon but if a cancer cure requires a vegetarian or raw vegan diet, I'll do it, and had been for 10 months at that point). We drove through traffic consisting of as many motorbikes as cars, Mali and Chati conversing in Thai with frequent use of cell phones and occasional talk with me in the back seat.

It turned out that they were looking for a vegetarian restaurant. I tried to assure them that most restaurants would surely have vegetables and I could order some sort of salad, but they wanted to please me and kept searching.

Finally a place called "Salada" caught Mali's eye and we circled around waiting for the guard to allow us to enter the parking structure. We entered at last, drove through the entire multi-level garage and came out where we started for lack of any empty spot. The guard was kind and waved us over to an off-street area and into a vacant spot and we walked to the restaurant.

This was a big sort of restaurant mall. In the middle is a lake with a big fountain and a wide walkway around it, and restaurants are ranged around the entire walkway. Salada has its own organic veggie garden, as I could see from a big mural. I ordered two veggie appetizers, expecting them to be small, and a salad, but the appetizers turned out to consist of 10 veggie rolls each plus sauce. So I had 3 meals in front of me plus a second salad that Mali had ordered for sharing with me. Meanwhile, Chati had finished his meal and time was hurrying along. So I got much of the lunch boxed up and later ate it for dinner on the plane back to Tao Garden.

The stem cell research doctor was Dr. Chongrak* and the stem cell clinic was on an upper floor of a very tasteful downtown building. I'll be honest and admit that before we got in the elevator, we passed through a lobby with a coffee bar. It displayed every kind of chocolate delight you can imagine and I didn't get past it unscathed. Ate that treat later on the plane too —- super quality chocolate mousse. What is it about chocolate that humanity loves so much?

Upstairs, two staff members met me with plates of fresh fruit and a tall glass of coconut milk and meat. What a hospitable country Thailand is! Dr. Chongrak was on his way and in the meantime, I chatted with one nurse and had my blood pressure and pulse taken. The IV was already set up.

---

* Not his real name

When Dr. Chongrak arrived, I lay on one of the beds and the nurse started preparing to put the IV line into my hand. I urged them to use my port. Dr. Chongrak explained that the nurse wasn't trained in using ports and I replied that it was very easy and she could learn right now. I asked them to remove the paper tape and Dr. Chongrak did. I saw his face when he took enough of it off to see the tube projecting from the port. His eyes lit up and he said, "Oh, this is very easy!" So he helped the nurse attach the stem cell IV –- or rather, he watched her do it, as she too could see how easy it is.

The IV took only 20 minutes to drip. He and I spent that time talking. He's a very quick-witted and enthusiastic man and fun to talk to. He told me that the 10 million stem cells came from a placenta that was donated by the mother of a happy, healthy baby. I asked him to thank her for me, which surprised him some, but I hope he does it. After the 20 minutes, he said,

"You must sleep now. You're a one-day-old baby."

Because of our lunch delay, it was now late in the day and I had just about 15 minutes to sleep before we rushed off to the airport. Our Tao Garden bus picked me up and I was in bed by about 11 pm. I slept through breakfast the next morning and much of the afternoon.

Second Stem Cell Treatment

The second stem cell treatment was on April 2, 2013. It was in a different Bangkok clinic but organized by the same doctor. I was met at the airport around 11:30 am by two different young people than last time – a man who drove the car and spoke middling English and a woman who spoke no English. They were both very kind and good-hearted, as Thai people tend to be. Knowing that I was supposed to be on a raw vegan diet, they drove to a vegetarian restaurant (there are no raw vegan restaurants) and we had an excellent meal before continuing on to the clinic. It offers many cosmetic procedures such as laser skin improvement and hair removal; stem cells are just one of the many offerings listed on their glass front wall.

My appointment was at 2 pm and we arrived about 1:45. I relaxed in the front waiting area and the two young people disappeared. Behind a high counter were two others working on computers and at one side was a small desk where differing numbers of young women clustered through the afternoon, doing I don't know what that involved some merriment.

At 3 pm, I asked one of them when my treatment would begin. She looked blank and waved over another woman who said,

"The stem cells are not here yet. They're on the way."

So I sat down again, reminding myself that Thai appointment times were perhaps merely suggestions rather than commitments. I recalled driving in the Dominican Republic where road signs and stop lights were regarded as mere suggestions. I lay down on a sofa-thing and dozed for a while and at 3:45, I sat up and saw my driver near the small desk.

"Are the stem cells here yet?"

He finished his texting and said,

"They're on the way. Won't be long."

"It's already been long!" I said, getting a bit irritated. "It's nearly two hours since my appointment time! Where's Dr. Chongrak?"

"Oh, he's in a meeting," he said, gesturing up the nearby staircase.

"Well, could you go and ask him when the stem cells will get here?" I was mindful that the treatment required some resting afterwards and was starting to think about catching my return flight and hopefully having dinner beforehand.

The young man went upstairs and didn't come back. At 4:15, I was now angry. I got up just as another man came down the stairs, evidently another doctor. He handed me a lime yogurt and said soothingly,

"The stem cells are on the way, Ma'am. Please just relax."

"No!" I said, determined now to get to the bottom of all this vagueness. Were the cells lost? Had the company forgotten to thaw them out the required three days previously and were they now frantically waving hair dryers over them? I had no clue and all the office people were keeping solemn faces, absorbed in their jobs.

The yogurt man had disappeared out the back way but my driver now appeared, texting someone.

"Please go upstairs and find out from Dr. Chongrak when these stem cells will get here," I said to him. "And don't disappear or I'll go up there myself and bust into his meeting!"

He went upstairs and after 7 minutes had not returned so I stomped up, thankful there was a banister to keep my balance. I found the meeting room door already open and Dr. Chongrak on the phone. A woman on the sofa said,

"Dr. Chongrak is angry now. He's talking to the company."

He hung up and looked at me.

"They don't know anything about it. They say they sent the cells at 2 pm and they don't know what has happened."

I thought about my expensive stem cells frizzling out in the hot Bangkok streets, worthless for treatment. It was now 4:40 pm. Do I stay in a hotel tonight? Change my return flight? Dr. Chongrak assured me that the cells were good for 48 hours in their packaging, regardless of Bangkok's weather. While he was soothing me with reassuring words, the phone rang and someone downstairs picked it up. The yogurt man came upstairs.

"The courier will be here shortly," he said. Right, I thought. Shortly in Thai time. But I went downstairs and waited some more and at 5 pm, a tall, sweating man stumbled in the door, plonked a box on the counter, got a paper signed, and hustled out before anyone said a word. Turned out his car had broken down in heavy traffic and he'd called someone to come and fix it. Apparently that person had been in no hurry. Or perhaps someone had had to drive off to get some new part or other.

At 5:01 pm, the nurses called me into the treatment room. One took off my shoes, one held open the bathroom door for a quick visit, one positioned the IV pole, another brought me a blanket and a cup of coffee, and one inserted the needle. She did it very skillfully, scarcely hurting at all. (I had had the port removed, not expecting to need any more IV treatments.) I thanked them all with real gratitude and big smiles. Dr. Chongrak came in to see how I was and we talked a bit.

- Ten million baby stem cells in the IV bag;

- Donated by a local mother of a healthy, happy baby;

- The placenta was kept for something else and the stem cells were taken from the umbilical cord;

- The previous stem cell treatment was probably the cause of my curly hair — my previously straight brown-grey hair is now growing back after chemo as curly brown hair;

- I didn't need to rest or sleep but could leave immediately for the airport as long as I slept a lot in the coming days.

As I was putting shoes on and gathering my things to leave and my driver was waiting, Dr. Chongrak disappeared and returned with a plastic bag of food.

"For your dinner!" he said proudly and put it down next to me. It contained an entire loaf of bread plus two containers of what looked like cheese and ham plus some sort of pasty-looking item with dark-colored contents (chocolate?). He had sent someone to a local bakery. I thanked him sincerely and again when he came out, talking on his cell phone, to wave goodbye as the car drove away.

We got to the airport in good time and after finding the gate and obtaining some free mayo from a kind attendant in the food court, I sat down to make my dinner sandwiches. The bread was whole wheat and in the little boxes were not slices of cheese or ham but little white bread sandwiches with the crusts cut off — one with a slice of bologna and one with a smear of tuna salad. A far cry from giant American sandwiches loaded with pickles, ketchup and multiples of everything. The pasty contained spinach.

Never mind. The plane was boarding so I packed up the food and later combined things with what the airline offered and the chocolate mousse and made a reasonable dinner considering I was traveling.

I was picked up at the Chiang Mai airport by one of our Tao Garden van drivers and delivered to my bungalow door about 11 pm. A long hot day and somewhat stressful, but with happy baby stem cells in my blood, I was content and slept long that night. (Narrative continues on p. 119)

More About Stem Cells

Stem cell research dates back to the 1950s and has become a fast-moving area. However, I've found it hard to get anything more than superficial information online. For example, nowhere can I find any site about administering stem cells via an intravenous line, the way my treatments were done.

Stem cells are undifferentiated, generic body cells with the potential of generating specific types of body cells while remaining generic themselves. The two kinds of stem cells are embryonic and adult stem cells.

- Embryonic Stem Cells

A baby in the womb grows by its embryonic stem cells forming differentiated daughter cells which go on to divide many times and form specific body organs such as eyes, muscles, and skin.

For medical purposes, these stem cells can be obtained from umbilical cord blood immediately after birth and from the placenta, the tissue connected to the baby's navel via the umbilical cord. No fetal death is involved. When these embryonic cells are harvested for medical treatments after the baby's birth, they are referred to as adult stem cells and known as HUCT cells – Human Umbilical Cord Tissue.

So when Dr. Chongrak referred to me as a "one-day-old baby", he was referring to the very young age of the cells I'd received; but they had not been taken directly from the baby, who was happily getting to know its family at home. They'd been taken from the donated placenta. In my second treatment, they were taken from the donated umbilical cord.

- Adult Stem Cells

Every adult has stem cells that are responsible for repair of damaged body tissue. They are found in many types of tissue, e.g. brain, bone marrow, skin, teeth, and skeletal muscle. They are not undifferentiated like embryonic stem cells but instead generate new cells for the type of tissue they're found in. So for example, bone marrow stem cells generate all the types of blood cells and follicular stem cells generate hair follicles.

Use of a patient's own stem cells for a treatment rather than donated cells eliminates the possibility of rejection.

While Waiting For Results

After two stem cell treatments, I had a waiting period ahead. Nobody could predict exactly how long it might take for the stem cells to do their good work; nor could they predict whether they would indeed dispose of my leukemia. Perhaps they'd attend to my impaired balance or hearing; perhaps all three issues or something else entirely. I was going to be pleased at whatever they did.

Meanwhile, my bungalow had no WIFI. So each day, I put my Mac laptop inside the walker seat with a book and personal stuff and carefully wheeled it to the juice bar or clinic. That way, I stayed in email touch with friends and my sons. When the walker seat tore from this daily weight, I balanced the laptop on top of the seat. But one day as I eased the walker down the step in my doorway, it slid off the seat and crashed onto the little stone porch. In that awful moment, I decided to find new lodging with WIFI. This MacBook Pro is a tough little thing and wasn't damaged by that fall, but any more such falls might be fatal.

Across the road from my driveway, facing sideways to overlook the rice fields, were three cottages among tall trees. The middle one was empty, I knew, and its property manager was Yang, the woman who owned and ran The Yellow House, along the road to the left of my driveway (Tao Garden was to the right). The Yellow House was a combination coffee shop and second-hand clothing shop. So I asked Yang if I could see inside that cottage.

"You like the hou," she said as we walked along the road to the gate. "Owner my good friend. She fik it for you, nie."

The metal gate was double-width and six feet high but tiny Yang pushed it open and we walked over the recently-laid sharp stones that did duty as a driveway. A path cut through assorted thorny bushes and rocks and arrived around at the front of the three houses, facing downhill the same direction we'd walked along the road from the Yellow House. The view was lovely: a great expanse of young green rice plants in their watery peace, clumps of big trees, and the brilliant magenta bougainvillea along the high gate and fence of a large house across the field. All under intense blue.

Yang went up the steps of the first house.

"Aren't we looking at the middle house?"

"That one taken. Thit one for you."

The middle one had trees shading it but this first one didn't. Yang jingled keys as she found the right one and we were inside. It was one main room with two big windows looking across the porch to the paddies. One had a desk in front of it. No chair. Something called a kitchen in the back with an old yellow cupboard like the one my mother had when I was little. Colored glass decorating the two top doors where plates and cups went, a bread compartment and drawers in the middle and storage at the bottom. With fresh paint, it would have been quite nice-looking and to me, evocative of good home-cooking smells from the wood-burning stove. To the right, an adequate-looking bathroom (shower only and hot water on demand, so no storage tank; that's a good way of doing hot water, in my experience). Queen bed on the left, a dresser and small closet. Cement floors.

"Could the owner provide some matting for the floor?" I asked, picturing one either side of the bed and one in the kitchen.

"She do that. No problem."

"How about blinds on these windows?"

"She do that."

"Could she provide a stove for the kitchen and a refrigerator? Also a counter to work on?"

"She do that. She fik everything how you want."

"An air conditioning unit? I think it would be pretty hot here with just that one fan and no trees giving shade."

"You shee. She do everything."

I asked her about the WIFI she had assured me the house had.

"WIFI in laht hou. He get new one nek month. He tell me not trong enough and new one coming." That last house was in deep shade, barely visible among its huge old trees.

As we went down the steps, I said, "Would the owner put a railing on these steps? My balance isn't very good so I need a railing to hold on to."

"Railing. I tell her. She good woman."

"Well, if the owner does those things, I'd like to try it," I said. Certainly a step up from my bungalow — not that I was upset about the bungalow other than no WIFI, but I felt I had to move on to a bigger place.

"I talk to owner tonight. You come to Yellow Hou and we look nekt week. OK?"

Meanwhile, I also asked Dr. Palo if he knew of any vacant cottages and he asked among the clinic staff and came up with one that sounded promising.

"Have you seen it?" I asked him.

"No. We can see it this afternoon if you like. I'll drive you there after work and we can go to dinner." He had the use of a Tao Garden car some days and when we went to dinner in Chiang Mai, various of his friends, visiting Thailand or resident there, would join us for a lot of talk and laughs and good Thai chow.

So late afternoon we drove towards the main Chiang Mai road, past Dr. Palo's house that he had inherited from Dr. Lodi when he left Tao Garden.

"Do you like that house Dr. Palo? It looks very private back among those trees."

"I love it!" he said, with feeling. "There's not a sound at night and I sit out on the verandah and relax after busy clinic days, and I think about nothing at all!" I grinned. I knew that pleasure, of silent solitude and no worries. I didn't know it often enough though.

He turned off the local road onto a village road and then onto another village road and there was the cottage. It sat up on a small rise with greenery around it and no close neighbors.

"Perfect location," said Dr. Palo. A group of women, probably residents of this village, Doi Saket, I thought, were clustered around an old truck, talking Thai a mile a minute. One of them turned and approached us as we got out of the car.

"Come. I show you," she said to me. Dr. Palo strolled over to the group where several men had now appeared. I surmised that renting a Doi Saket house to a Westerner was a bit of an event. It brought money to the community.

We went up the steps and Ting, as she introduced herself, ushered me in. A gentle breeze filled the house as I looked around the main room. Queen bed on the left with refrigerator next to it instead of a nightstand. It was almost an open-plan layout and as I walked into the "kitchen", I saw the source of the gentle breeze. There was no wall on the side or most of the back of this area. A metal sink stood at the end with a cold-water tap and trees behind it; a counter ran along the back, stark against the back-yard weeds; and a cabinet stood against what back wall there was.

"Will the owner be putting walls in here?" I asked Ting.

She looked a bit uncertain, as if she hadn't understood my English.

"Is there hot water?"

"In bathroom. Hot water here." She showed me the hose running up one wall with a shower head on its end. "Plenty hot water." It was the on-demand arrangement again.

The bathroom sink had one tap only. Cold.

Well, Thailand is a hot country and I told myself that perhaps I should consider living with no kitchen hot water or walls. I'd seen other local houses apparently with only partial exterior walls. Perhaps it was a centuries-old tradition. So I said, "What about some fly screens on these two wall areas?"

"Owner do that. I think."

There was no back door. No air conditioning unit but what use would it be with missing walls?

"Fly creen. You live here?" asked Ting. I told her I'd think about it. She seemed to regard it as a fine house and I didn't want to seem rude.

Dr. Palo drove us into Chiang Mai talking of this and that and me appreciating my old bungalow a bit more. A few days later, I walked over to the three houses I'd looked at with Yang. It was Wednesday and the Yellow House was closed and Yang not there, but I thought I could at least see if the owner had installed a railing on those front steps. She had. I used it to mount the steps and peer through the front windows. No matting. No window blinds. No kitchen amenities as far as I could see.

A few days later, I decided to move to Chiang Mai. I got online and found some rentals and ended up taking a three-bedroom, two-story house in a gated community. From one housing extreme to another. There was a nice yard, a big sliding gate I could lock, a balcony. The woman who showed it to me lived in a similar house behind this one. She had an English husband and together they ran a housing rental business. She told me about the neighbor on my right, a man called Hahn who was freshly retired back to Thailand after living and working in Phoenix, AZ. So I had bilingual neighbors and good security and I went about moving in with pleasure.

A day or two before I left Tao Garden, I was having lunch at a table with others, Howie included, the man who had told me about the Dark Room. After that Dark Room week was over and the participants showed up again in the dining room, I had asked him and some others how it had been. They had all responded rather vaguely that it was good but seemed reluctant to go into any detail. I'm sure they had all encountered aspects of themselves that didn't bear much discussion with relative strangers so I didn't press them.

"Jen, I hear you're moving into Chiang Mai soon," Howie said.

"Yes, it's going to be quiet around here. Looks like most of the Dark Room people have already left."

"The season will be over soon," Howie said. "The Master goes traveling in the off-season."

"Does he travel to Germany?"

"Most years he does. He gives talks – in other European countries too. It generates interest in Tao Garden and brings more people here for classes. Since you're moving to Chiang Mai, I wonder if you'd like to know about Tim. She drives a taxi."

"I certainly will be needing a taxi, Howie, so yes, who's Tim?"

"When I had my restaurant in Phuket, I couldn't find organic supplies in that area — good coconut oil, organic rice and fresh produce etc. So I hired Tim to find them up here. She knows all the health food stores in Chiang Mai."

I gave him a big grin. He knew I'd been through bad cancer times and had been a raw vegan. "Give me Tim's phone number right now!"

"She's a capable woman," he said, jotting it down. "She packaged everything up and had it shipped to my restaurant every time I called her. She's a Chiang Mai native."

I put the piece of paper in my pocket. "I'm going to like Tim," I said. "Thanks. Have a good flight tomorrow. I'm glad to have met you, Howie."

We clasped hands. I got up to organize my walker and he left to start packing for his Germany flight.

A New Thai Friend

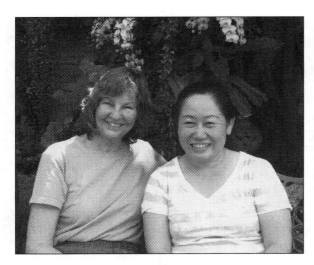

Jen and Tim

---Photo by Unknown Passer-by

I did indeed like Tim.* To stock my new kitchen, I soon needed a thorough shopping trip and I arranged with Tim over the phone that she'd be at my place at 10 am.

She arrived at 9:55am in a big yellow van, an official taxi. Not all Chiang Mai taxis are official. But since Tim's was, she had permission to wait in line at the airport, picking up new arrivals. She did more than just drive them to their hotel. Talking to them, she'd piece together what their interests were and how much time they had, and then spent it showing them the sights.

There are many one-lane streets in Chiang Mai but they're used as two-lane streets. Somebody just backs up if necessary. As a Chiang Mai native, Tim knew every back

---

* Not her real name, but she did have a male name per Western names.

street and obscure shop and all the tourist attractions, and she gave cheery and efficient service. If traffic was slow going by one route, she darted along a narrow side street and took another route.

We became friends. The first day, she decided where to take me and we turned into a stony parking lot lined with assorted shops, one of which offered organic products.

"I know this place!" I said. "It's the Mosquito Shop!"

Tim looked at me quizzically.

"The floor's full of mosquitoes. I was wearing sandals and I got bitten the whole time we were here. Dr. Palo drove three of us here to get some anti-cancer items. I swore I'd never come here again."

"Well, we here," said Tim, laughing and looking at my feet, wearing sandals again. "No need for walker Jen," she said, holding out her arm.

"All right, I'll try it again. It did have some good stuff." I grinned and took hold of her arm, fanny pack safe around my waist. I stepped carefully over the broken cement and weeds and at the door, picked up a plastic basket. The shop was laid out sideways with a center double-sided shelf and shelves lining front, left side and back walls and the checkout counter on the right side.

"What you need?" she asked.

I consulted my list and peered at the nearest shelf. All labels were in Thai.

"Well, some coconut oil, chia seeds, almonds, cashews, tahini, coconut milk, curry powder …"

Tim was already at the left end of the shop with several items in her hands. We filled the basket easily and I crossed many things off my list. My feet did get bitten in the Mosquito Shop but it was worth it for the good items I could buy there.

There were five health food shops in Chiang Mai, counting the Vegetarian Society, a restaurant with a shop in one area. There was also the Rimping Meechok supermarket which caters to both Thais and Europeans and offers many organic and non-typical items. "Rimping" means "close to the Ping river", a fairly large river we crossed each time we drove between my house and Old Town. Meechok is the name of the area. We went to that shop most often because it was biggest.

Tim stands about as high as my shoulders but she was like my little second mother and she started educating me. First she'd have me read items from my list. Then while we looked for them, she'd say things like,

"You try thee avocado? Grown in Thailand. Cheaper." I love avocados.

"You want corn? Very fresh." I did at first but stopped after I learned that it was a standard GMO crop (genetically modified).

"You try durian?" Durians are huge heavy fruit with thick skins covered in big sharp spikes. They're highly nutritious but the best way of buying them, I thought, was in packaged pieces. Once cut, they smell like dirty feet. Dr. Palo loved them. Once when he was driving the three of us cancer patients at Tao Garden to go shopping, he spotted a man selling cut durian on the street and he promptly pulled over and double parked. He wanted to introduce durian to us all. As soon as we got out of the car we could smell it but he urged us on enthusiastically.

"Forget the smell, ladies. It tastes wonderful and it's so good for you!"

Coming from our doctor, that carried weight. So we all bought a chunk and sat on a stone ledge nearby to munch and we did all like it. Once you get the taste of it, the smell becomes less prominent. So sometimes shopping with Tim I bought a packet of cut pieces and was always pleased.

I also began educating her about shopping for a cancer patient.

"I love mangos, Tim, but I can't eat them. They're too sweet." I was avoiding tropical fruit because of its high fructose content.

"Tim, that almond milk is not good for someone with cancer. Here's the ingredient list. See, it has 24 grams of sugar. This one has just eight grams."

She didn't read English as she had learned to speak it by listening to her taxi passengers and talking to them. But she'd remember the brand, the look of it, and know it was too sugary.

She remembered what items I'd bought before and checked with me if they weren't on my list.'

"You need more aloe joo?" "Chinee cabbage?"

So we worked our way through the Rimping Meechok supermarket often, with me pushing the cart as a walker and Tim flitting around, reading labels to me, finding things, and getting answers from store employees. Sometimes there were special deals where the customer would be given a free gift if they bought several of a certain item. The first one was dark chocolate. If I bought 3 packets of 85% dark chocolate, the store would give me a free coffee mug. I gave it to Tim. That deal lasted several weeks and Tim was happy to get a set of mugs while I was happy to buy lots of chocolate. There were other such deals too and it became a game, finding them. I ate too much chocolate. But I told myself, "Eighty-five percent dark chocolate has very little sugar. And it's a superfood and has good nutrients like iron and magnesium and copper, and lots of fiber. And the little bit of caffeine won't make me miss any sleep. And it's a big antioxidant and I can't get too much of those."

I thought that was all persuasive. It is all true but when you like chocolate so much that you eat an entire bar after dinner, you're on a slippery slope – the sugar adds up and you ingest tons of calories. Chocolate is one of my comfort foods though. In this long cancer slog and always living alone, I appreciated comfort food. In my wicked days living in Denver, I had bought many chocolate desserts (mousse or cake or brownie), with whipped cream (real cream), nuts, and sometimes ice cream too. Scrumptious! But those sinful times are gone. Now I suffer the angel of water to baptize me within. ☺ (pp. 63-64).

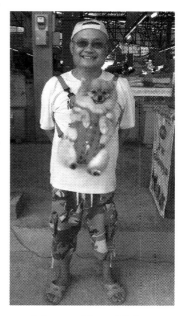

When we got back to my house, Tim would take the key, which I left in the little tray in the console, unlock the door while I got myself and the walker out of the car, and help me carry the bags in. She offered to help me put them away too, but I preferred to do that myself, first washing the vegetables and then storing them in my green vegetable bags which keep them fresh for longer. I paid her gladly each time, happy with all the help she gave me and all the fun we had.

My neighbor, Hahn

Photo by Jen Kimberley

127

A Good Neighbor

Hahn, on the right side of my house, as you walk out the door, was a retired accountant. He had planted tons of flowers in his front yard, a modest size like mine and all the houses in this development except the few grand ones, and it was a riot of color. Annuals and perennials grew along the front fence and orchids hung from the trees and fence. Orchids flourish in Thailand, growing there naturally, and every front yard that I saw featured several, including mine.

Hahn was a cheerful man with a square face and big smile. He stood a bit higher than my shoulders. He had a tiny dog, a Pomeranian, and carried it everywhere in a baby carrier on his chest, or in the front basket of his bicycle. In my first week in this new house, I didn't see him. I was busy unpacking and getting settled in. The house had no washing machine or dryer. In Thailand, I never saw an electric clothes dryer; most people have a big clothes rack, a tall four-wheeled structure with many rails, that you can push into a sunny place or shady as you prefer. Mine was in the carport and I had noticed early on that it was missing a wheel. One day in my second week there, I saw that it had its four wheels intact. I also noticed that the big front gate was much easier to open and close.

"I think Hahn fixed them," said my agent, who had popped over to give me the gate key.

So I approached Hahn's big gate and saw him coming out his front door, dog squirming in his arms. He put the doggie, trembling with excitement, in his bike basket and unlocked his gate.

"Hello Hahn, my name is Jen."

"I know," he said. The dog started barking in its squeaky soprano voice. "He's impatient. He wants me to get going."

"Where are you riding to?"

"Going to the market to get dinner," he said. "I'll take you some time if you like." Hahn's carport held a nice looking compact car.

"I would like that. Did you fix my clothes rack?"

"Yes. That wheel's been off for months. Nobody's been living there since Ling moved out."

"The yard does need some mowing and pruning," I said.

"Your gate was stiff too so I gave it some oil."

"I noticed. Thanks so much!" The dog was bouncing and barking. I held out my hand and it gave me a perfunctory lick.

"This is Ritchie."

"Hello, little Ritchie fur ball," I crooned. His fur was so thick I could barely feel his body shape. "You're in for an exciting ride. Well I'll see you later, Hahn."

He left his gate open and waved as he rode off, Ritchie quiet now and super alert to the fast moving smells.

Hahn was a fabulous neighbor and we became friends. Being so familiar with both Thailand and America, he knew what to teach me and enjoyed doing it. We did drive to the market some afternoons – a noisy crowded place with a cacophony of smells from all the meats and fish being cooked. Each hot food stall had a spinning device overhead, several spokes or strings that turned incessantly to keep flies away. Long electric cords slithered and draped their way to outlets I never did locate. There were soups and fresh vegetables and fruit and every kind of edible product – except durian, I noticed. So no dirty feet smell interfered with the dinner aromas. I bought some tasty soup many days, some nameless concoctions that looked (and were) delicious, and vegetables from the King's Project.

The King of Thailand has an organic vegetable farm, or at least minimally sprayed. He's an old man now and very loved by the Thai people. The Rimping supermarket sold his vegetables too but at steeper prices than our neighborhood market. I bought no meat or fish as I was being a vegetarian, still in the aftermath of raw veganism.

Hahn also took me to his laundry. It was close by on the main road that went to Doi Saket and Tao Garden, and was run by two industrious women, one in front dealing with customers and sorting clothes and the other in back doing ironing. Each week I gave them my laundry stuffed in a plastic bag and a day or two later retrieved it, each item neatly ironed and folded and with a precise list of each item and its cost taped to the bag. I ran a tab with them.

A Paw Paw Partnership

One day, on Hahn's side of my house where there were bushes galore, a passion fruit vine and a tall tree, I noticed a half-rotten paw paw on the ground. I squinted up against the intense blue and saw many in a cluster – my paw paw tree was bearing fruit. But how to pick them, so high up? The tree stood exactly outside the second floor spare room window and its fruit was at window level. But all the houses in this development had fixed cast iron grillwork over the windows, the spaces too narrow for a paw paw to fit through.

Hahn and I went to work. First he used his ladder (my wobbly balance put ladders beyond my ability at this time), and for that first cluster of fruit, he was able to reach and dislodge it. I stood below and caught each one as he dropped it. The lowest ones ripened first and ripeness worked its way up the big cluster. For the top dozen or so his ladder wasn't tall enough so he attached a bucket to a long stick and upstairs, I reached through the window grill to dislodge each paw paw and standing on the ladder, he caught them in the bucket – a short drop so they weren't bruised. A few weeks later, the second cluster was higher still. The last dozen or so were too high for me to reach through the window, so I used a long wooden spoon to nudge and Hahn caught. Sometimes if I was out, he had his cleaning lady, Tang (now our mutual cleaning lady), reach through the window.

I offered paw paws to them both and Tang accepted happily, having several children to feed. Hahn didn't want the work of peeling them so I peeled and cut them for him, leaving a covered bowlful at his front door if he was out.

Papaya Leaf Tea For Cancer

There are "papayas" and there are "paw paws". In America, papayas (Latin name *Asimina trebola*) are common but in my years of living there, I never saw a pawpaw, which are much bigger. I believe they grow in the South though. The leaves are different from those of a papaya tree and the tree shape is different, although to me, anyway, the fruit tastes the same. My paw paw tree was *carica papaya*, the type with large fruit.

In one of the health food stores one day, a fellow customer I was talking to said that papaya leaf tea was a good cancer treatment. The store had some (using paw paws, *carica papaya*) so I bought a bottle and started drinking it that evening. Then I read online about it and found that while it is anti-cancer and is being studied further; and it does increase red cell counts, which would probably be good for most people, one thing it also does is raise platelet levels. My form of leukemia raises platelet levels already so papaya leaf tea would be risky. Platelets being necessary for blood clotting, we need a certain number of them, but too many could form a clot in the bloodstream, aside from any break in the skin, and such a clot could travel to the heart or brain, causing a heart attack or stroke, respectively. I poured out the tea. But for someone with a tumorous cancer, it would be well worth trying.

Getting Some Wheels

As a cancer patient, I still needed exercise as now I had no access to Tao Garden's gym or salt swimming pool. I started taking longer walks in the housing development. The streets were quiet and safe; the entrance was guarded and even at night there were guards patrolling. The streets were also pretty new, with smooth surfaces, unlike Chiang Mai's Old Town streets which were composed of broken cement, missing bricks, sudden little drop-offs, and trees that required you to walk on the road with the alarming traffic. So I walked in my neighborhood and got to know many of the dogs, fenced in all day while their owners were at work and bored out of their doggy skulls.

There was a (chlorine) swimming pool nearby and I walked there many days and swam laps, allowing for children's games if I arrived after school was out.

One day, Hahn said,

"What if you had a tricycle, Jenny?"

I saw my small brother pedaling and puffing on his tiny tricycle, his dinky – as a girl, I hadn't been allowed to have a dinky. I must have looked bemused.

"An adult tricycle. They have them at the bike shop where I went yesterday. They have a big basket between the back wheels and a regular one on the handlebars. You could bring stuff home from the Market."

Suddenly it was the perfect idea.

"Yes! You're a genius, Hahn! Can you drive me there today?"

"Well, let me negotiate for you first. I'll go tomorrow and see if they have a nice one and get the price down for you."

So a few days later, I bought one and Hahn had arranged for the shop owner to buy it back when I left Thailand. Now I could range further afield. I hopped on it and hopped right off again! I couldn't ride even one yard, such a panic I felt at having the world suddenly move quickly. It destroyed my leisurely visual cues. All through 2012 I grew used to the world bouncing with each movement I made —- like living on a boat in choppy waters. After pushing the walker for a year, I had graduated to a walking stick and now proceeded at a stately pace.

But the trike swept me back to square one as regards getting around. I practiced and after a week or so, I could ride the length of my little street, all of five houses long, and back. Then I could venture to the swimming pool or jogging park, six or seven blocks and back. Next was riding around any and all of the nice flat streets in this development. My appearance around each corner brightened up the dull days of lots of dogs behind their fences. Some of them grew quiet as they got to know me and I would stop to stroke their lonely heads and talk to them. Sometimes a free-roaming dog brightened my day till I pedaled far enough away from his territory.

One day I got brave and rode out of the development, turning left into the surrounding village. The road had been resurfaced because of another housing development starting further along. After that point, the pot holes were more than I could handle, but this was a pleasant trip, the houses unpretentious, dogs otherwise occupied, hens pecking happily in the dust, and the temple gleaming gold in the sun behind its wall with Buddha statues. (Continued on p. 136)

Cancer and Exercise

Our bodies are made to move. Anyone who lives a sedentary lifestyle (like writers) is stressing their body even though they're quiet all day.

Moving the Lymph

Lymph drainage, part of the body's natural detoxification, depends on muscle movement. Muscles contracting and relaxing stimulate nearby lymph vessels to move their contents along. With no heart pumping lymph, body movement stimulates forward flow and valves prevent backflow. Lymph carries waste products from body cells, filters some out in lymph nodes, and delivers the lymph to venous blood via tiny capillaries. (See pp. 64-69 for more on lymph.)

Moving the Blood

Our heart pumps arterial blood out to the body and it travels in ever-smaller vessels until the tiniest ones are wide enough only for one cell at a time, single file. This way, each red cell delivers oxygen and the plasma delivers nutrients to the body cells bordering that single-lane pathway. At the same time, carbon dioxide and other waste products are moved from the body cells into the blood. Now the blood is carrying these back to the heart, traveling in ever-larger vessels as they all join the large veins that deliver the venous blood to the heart.

All this venous blood movement needs body movement to operate well. Our muscles contain lots of little veins and contraction and relaxation of that muscle tissue compresses and releases the veins, thus pushing the blood along.

What Sort of Exercise?

A daily walk would be good, about half an hour long. Dancing, bike riding, horse riding, roller blading, ice skating, -- anything that moves your whole body and increases your heartbeat moderately. When the body exerts itself in these ways, the cells are working faster to use nutrients and dispose of waste products; so the blood must move more quickly to take care of that, and the heart therefore pumps faster. But you don't want to overdo it such that the body gets exhausted and can't dispose of all the extra toxins and dead cells released by cancer treatments.

Other Ways That Exercise Helps With Cancer

By increasing blood flow, exercise increases the circulation of white cells in the blood, enabling them to find and destroy more cancer cells.

Traditionally, oncologists have urged rest, not exercise, for cancer patients undergoing conventional treatments. We need more research on how exercise affects cancer but some studies have already shown that regular exercise:

- o Helps to lower estrogen levels and therefore reduces recurrence of breast cancer;

- o Triggers apoptosis (death of sick or old cells);

- o Helps reduce body fat – this has been correlated with reduced numbers of tumors;

- o Maybe lowers the risk of prostate cancer by lowering testosterone levels.

As with all health issues, it is important to listen to your body. It might need a rest period or gentler exercise; or it might be eager for more muscle movement. A gym membership and even a personal trainer could be excellent, providing many ways of exercising and strengthening muscles in the right order so as to avoid injuries. Imagine the benefits if we had oncologists who worked with fitness trainers who devised a safe customized program for each of us.

Leaving Thailand

When I had moved to this housing development, it had been May 2013. My stem cell treatments, for which I had come to Thailand, had been in February and April. I had asked the doctor how long it would take to see results and he had said nobody knew. Nobody can predict exactly what the stem cells will do in any particular person. They are known to be capable of curing leukemia, which is why I had these treatments, but that isn't a certain result. So I was waiting an unknown time to see unknown results, if any. Meanwhile, I liked Thailand and was happy to stay there, and I ended up staying for 14 months.

In March, 2014 I felt it was time to move on. It seemed that those baby stem cells had done their job – they had fixed my hair. It was now a little browner and a little wavy. Fixing leukemia was apparently not on their To Do list. Not that I was ungrateful for the hair improvement. But I felt that it was time to figure out what to do next for the cancer. Dr. Lodi was busy with clinic development and Dr. Palo was in Bangkok getting ready to return to Zambia. So I had no cancer doctor.

My last day was a bit chaotic. I had already given my computer desk to Tim. She has two young boys and the older one had started to learn computer skills at school. He wanted his own computer and Tim was saving up for it. So the desk and surge protector went to him. I'd also given her my walker. She supports her mother as well as her two boys, with a little help from her husband, and her mother apparently had severe osteoporosis. The walker enabled her to stand upright instead of bent over at a right angle.

Because of a prior commitment to show some tourists the sights, Tim was unable to drive me to the airport on my last day but she sent a taxi-driving friend whom I hadn't met. He arrived an hour early with his wife and young daughter and I was running late. So while I hurried up and down the stairs gathering my last bits and pieces and hoping the suitcases weren't too heavy, he and his family sat in the living room watching. They spoke no English. Hahn was there too so they spoke to him a little. Our cleaning lady Tang was there too, working on Hahn's house but also hanging around my house doing nothing in particular. When I started clearing out the kitchen cupboards and refrigerator, I realized I still had a lot of usable stuff, though I'd already given a lot to Tim. Then I realized what everyone was waiting for: food items I couldn't take with me.

I didn't mind. Feeling like Santa Claus, I gave bottles and boxes of good stuff to the taxi driver's wife and her dignified gratitude was moving. She and her daughter packed it all into paper bags I supplied. Tang got her share too. Thai women work hard and I was glad to help. Hahn helped me with packing:

"Did you get everything from the bathrooms?"

"Anything still in the bedroom?"

"I don't think these suitcases are too heavy."

"Want me to do a run-through?"

Not too far off punctual, the taxi was loaded up and I said goodbye to Hahn. And a heartfelt thank you. What a good neighbor he'd been!

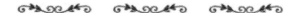

Memorandum

✓ Stem cells are generic cells that can produce specific types of body cells, e.g. heart or skin cells;

✓ We all have our own adult stem cells and they can be used to treat health problems;

✓ Baby stem cells can be obtained from an umbilical cord or a placenta when a new mother donates them;

✓ Stem cells can cure leukemia and other conditions but there is no guarantee that they will.

✓

✓

✓

Chapter 7: Getting Some Testing

It was lateish at night in March 2014 when my plane landed at Denver airport but a friend, John, was there to pick me up. John (not his real name) was an extremely good handyman and had worked on my house as well as my friend Sue's. I immediately went into culture shock: I could read the road signs! I understood everything John said! His driver's seat was to my left, not to my right, and he drove on the right (wrong) side of the road, not the left side. It was a familiar drive from the airport to downtown Denver but it seemed remote also, like something I'd once dreamed. As we approached Sue's house down I-25, the main north/south freeway through Denver, that familiar-but-remote feeling intensified and when Jim unlocked the front door and I entered Sue's living room, I had to sit down. She had painted all the interior walls, giving her décor a rich, colorful feel instead of the neutral feel I recalled.

Sue was still away for the weekend and once John had brought in my luggage and made sure I didn't need him to do anything else, he left and I sat there, at home but a foreigner.

And there was Sue's piano. I looked at the music books on top of it and started playing from one. It was a beginner's book and I'd had about five years of lessons in the past but I shied away from thinking how long ago that had been. From lack of playing, I was now a beginner again myself, with arthritic fingers as well. I played a little piece from the Anna Magdalena Bach book (written by Bach for his second wife, who was learning to play keyboard). Bach's music is always healing to me, whether it's buoyant secular music or heart-rending Easter music. It repairs my energy. I played several Bach pieces. Downstairs in the basement was my bedroom that I'd slept in previously for a few months when I'd lost my rental situation and hadn't yet found a house to buy. After enough Bach I stumbled down the stairs and fell into the ready-made bed. Sue is a generous and thoughtful hostess.

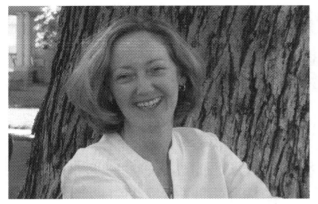

Sue Hunt, warm and supportive friend
and generous hostess.

---Photo by Jen Dundee

When she returned from her skiing trip, we got to talking and catching up and determining how I could best be a housemate for her. She has worked for many years at the phone company, weathering two company takeovers and being retrained twice for new work. I'd left Denver in 2010; now three-and-a-half years later, we were both different people to some extent. With no car, I'd be staying at home a lot so I took on a few chores to lighten her load.

One was emptying the compost bucket. Sue grows vegetables every summer; I tried to do some weeding too but my balance was still off. Bending over I'd lose my precarious sense of "Up" and could easily fall. Another was care for her new kitten, Benjy – a little orange cat that we picked up one evening early on as she had lost both her older cats. One had died of old age and the other had escaped into the neighborhood and never been found. Later, she obtained a second kitten and I had a doubly delightful job. I also helped keep the kitchen clean and folded laundry.

In my ten previous Denver years, Sue had been my dancing sister. She still went dancing as often but I had to stay home. My balance seemed to be returning, but very slowly. Each day I worked on this Saga, read about cancer, and mused about what to do next, where to live, and how to deal with the CML without taking any chemo pill. It occurred to me (belatedly) that with leukemia, arthritis, early cataracts both left and right, hearing loss, balance loss, and persistent diarrhea or constipation, I should learn more about my own health.

There are hundreds of tests one can have to determine specific things about health – vitamin or mineral deficiencies, food allergies, blood levels of this or that, urine tests, spit tests – I had never known where to start. So I'd put the idea aside. Now, kitten on my lap, I started a new round of online reading and video watching. Some of the things I learned are:

1. Every leukemia patient has a heavy metal load.

   o Well, in this toxic world many think we all have a heavy metal load. I'd had a urine test for heavy metals done in the Arizona clinic that had shown seven of the 20 absent, seven more "within reference", and six "outside reference", meaning too high. Looked like I was rather ahead in this particular game.

2. Melatonin, a hormone produced by the brain's pineal gland, increases in darkness and decreases when light enters the eyes. It's often used as a sleep aid supplement. However it does other things too, one of which is raising the white blood cell levels. This could be excellent for some people but leukemia increases the white cells to blood-cluttering levels so melatonin would not be good for a leukemia patient.

   o I'd been taking melatonin for two years so now I stopped it.

3. The body has "pathways" for accomplishing its processes whereby a series of actions leads to a goal being accomplished, such as a food being digested or a skin injury being healed. If one of the actions in the pathway fails to happen, health problems ensue. The liver has detoxification pathways and they're in two phases called simply Phase I and Phase II. Phase I prepares toxins and makes them available and Phase II has them escorted out of the body.

   o From reading Hulda Clark and having my liver palpated every doctor visit for eight years, I knew how crucial good liver function is. In Thailand, I'd let go of my resistance to coffee enemas and done one every day for ten months. I resolved to continue them to make sure this super-important organ did not get overworked. (See pp. 62-64)

4. You can overdo things with supplements and get yourself overdosed. Hyperthyroidism would be as much of a problem as hypothyroidism. Some of its symptoms are fatigue, nervousness, heart palpitations and weight loss, all from the body having too much thyroid hormone.

   o I stopped taking the thyroid hormone supplement I'd been on for two years, deciding to get a thyroid test.

I read more and the information out there was endless. It was time to switch from general information to specific facts about my own health or lack thereof.

Some Helpful Tests

Sue is a health-conscious person and she took me to a medical office where we both ordered a variety of tests. I ordered 12 and here are some that would be helpful for many people:

Vitamin D	Cancer incidence is associated with vitamin D deficiency and studies so far have shown that the right amounts of it can trigger cancer cell death (apoptosis) and reduce blood vessel formation to tumors.
Fasting Glucose	Since sugar in the form of high fructose corn syrup is in virtually all processed foods, high blood sugar levels have become common and are leading to higher incidence of diabetes as well as cancer. This test measures your amount of blood sugar when you've had no recent food.
C-reactive protein*	An inflammation marker to start getting a picture of body-wide disease (e.g. cancer, arthritis, cataracts, candida). Inflammation underlies all disease. There are other inflammation markers too.
A stool test	To detect the intestinal presence of assorted bacteria and molds and digestive residues such as sugar, fat, and water; also to assess mal-digestion by measuring the presence of pancreatic enzymes and bile acids; and other items including some you can specially request.

---

* The "C" in this name dates from research done in the 1930s on the *pneumococcus* bacterium where two elements of it were known when a third one was found; it was named Fraction C, being the third. Later more research led to its name being C-Reactive Protein. It's a tiny protein that's present during illness and disappears when the illness does.

A food allergy test	We can live for years eating foods we're allergic to and never realize it. We assign other reasons for our digestive troubles, headaches, fatigue, skin eruptions and other symptoms. These problems are named food sensitivities to distinguish them from the more dramatically obvious allergies like hives or breathing difficulty.
Complete Blood Count	This gives an overview of your blood component levels. If your white cells, red cells or platelets are outside their normal ranges, further testing would be advisable to discover why.

The above is a very small list of what's available. What tests you need depends on your particular history and current troubles and your doctor or naturopath will know where to start.

A Different Kind of Blood Test

In April, 2014, I went to a weekend workshop in Chicago where there was a nurse with a dark field microscope. She sat to one side and one by one we all went to get a small finger prick and see our blood up on the large projection screen. Off to the other side was a PEMF machine (Pulsed ElectroMagnetic Field Therapy). The idea was to look at your blood before and after a PEMF treatment to see how the treatment affected it.

- Before PEMF, my blood looked much the way it had a year previously in Thailand. (I'll post the photo at jenkimberley.com; its resolution is too low for print output.) The red cells were still clumped together though there weren't as many dysfunctional white cells. As we watched on the big screen, there was little movement, just sluggish red cell movement.

- After PEMF, there was lots of movement. The red cells were much more separated and were dancing around on the microscope slide. Being outside the live bloodstream, they had nowhere to go but they were going there energetically. The nurse timed it and it lasted seven minutes; then they subsided into the previous sluggish movement. She said that in more healthy blood, they would have danced for more like 30 minutes, having more energy in their stores. The white cells were still inactive, the leukemic cells large and dysfunctional, and the smaller normal white cells dotted around in between them.

The PEMF machine is very simple to use:

1. Make sure the frequency knob is at its lowest position;

2. Place the coil on your body where you want treatment and turn the frequency knob to whatever setting you want, whether slower and stronger or faster and weaker;

3. Turn it on.

Number 1 above is important. Later on in Germany at Arcadia Klinik (see Chapter 8), I used the PEMF machine every evening after dinner. One night I was sleepy and careless. I placed the coil around my head, hoping to help my hearing and balance improve, and turned it on without checking the frequency knob's position. I about flew out of the chair! It was on a high setting and the impact was huge and the sound loud, close around my ears. Once was enough to learn that lesson. Setting it low to start with allows you to increase it comfortably to whatever level is best. However, even on the highest setting, it causes no damage in the body, just possible discomfort. Remember to set the machine on Low when you leave.

At this workshop, I heard about that Arcadia Klinik mentioned above and how it offers a treatment that's unavailable in many countries: hyperthermia. After I studied the clinic's website, the idea grew in me that hyperthermia could be the hitherto missing treatment that I needed. Seeing the sluggish white and red blood cells in the microscope suggested to me that my entire immune system might be dormant. If I spent a few weeks there, I could have further testing, good medical advice, a good anti-cancer diet since it's a residential clinic, and a fresh chance to chase away my leukemia. When I returned to Sue's house, I applied at Arcadia and was accepted. They were right then in the process of moving from their premises in Kassel, a large busy town, to larger premises in Bad Emstal, a small, quiet spa town. They suggested I wait a few weeks so I booked a plane ticket two weeks away and in great excitement started packing.

(Narrative continued on p. 144)

Benefits of PEMF

Pulsed Electro-Magnetic Frequencies (PEMF) are delivered quietly, easily, comfortably and inexpensively. If you are wondering how you can best improve your immunity and strengthen your body to deal with cancer of any kind, a PEMF unit is a fine answer.

PEMF increases blood flow, bringing more oxygen to body cells and boosting cell metabolism. We have lost a lot of the natural electro-magnetic energy from planet earth that people took for granted years ago. According to ongoing measurements of Earth's magnetic field, it now measures at 0.5 gauss instead of the estimated 5.0 gauss of about 4,000 years ago. And our 0.5 gauss is distorted by legions of mobile phones, satellite signals, and all the electrical vibrations of our high-tech lives.

The pulsed electro-magnetic energy of a PEMF treatment gives the body fuel to create cellular energy and this helps us heal ourselves not just of cancer, but of all degenerative diseases. We have something over 70 trillion cells, all with specific jobs to accomplish, and by giving them extra magnetic energy, PEMF provides a lot of benefits. It will:

o   Kill cancer cells;

o   Stimulate production of DNA and RNA;

o   Increase calcium distribution and absorption, which would help strengthen bones and joints;

o   Stimulate endorphin release;

o   Stimulate cellular repairs;

o   Increase collagen production for better skin elasticity;

o   Speed up detoxification of both organs and cells

It can also reduce swelling and its associated pain and provide many other benefits too numerous to list here. There's no limit on how many PEMF treatments anyone can have – several a day if you like.

---From a blog written by Jen Kimberley

Energy Work #4: Havingness

You might have heard about people who pine after winning the lottery so they can buy a bigger house, for example, and one day they do win. Then three months later, the money's gone and they're still crouching in their small house. When it actually came to buying the big house, their havingness failed them. The money was scattered around on things they didn't particularly need or want like cruises, furniture, parties or things the kids clamored for. They couldn't allow themselves to have a big house and so they allowed all else to take priority.

Another sign of low havingness is chronic cynicism. When a person habitually rejects good ideas or good news or receives them with disbelief or skepticism and immediately points out possible downsides, it's because they carry a chronically low havingness. An example I encounter:

"Cure cancer? Nah. The doctors can't cure it so how could we do it ourselves?"

Their faces express disbelief with underlying discomfort and desire for it not to be true. Accepting this truth would cause them to have to adjust something in themselves and they shy away from such a prospect.

Kinds of Havingness

There is general havingness and specific havingness. A person might seem to always be "lucky"; life always seems to go their way, things drop into their lap. That person has high general havingness. They can allow good things to happen and they don't get bogged down in guilt because others haven't got so many good things happening; or in fear that if things are so good, surely they'll crash soon; or in self-abnegation, telling themselves, "I don't deserve this good fortune, this is not right." They accept good things happening as part of life.

We can also have a havingness level for anything specific in life: for cash, for friendships, for a slim body, vibrant health, vacation time – you can surely think of many more. We might have high havingness for social status but low havingness for close friends. Or high havingness for physical health but low havingness for money. Or the reverse.

Whatever havingness levels we have, we can raise them. It's like any other energy work: we see it the way we want it, then clear out any obstacles to its manifesting.

To Raise Your Havingness

Get comfortable in your energy work chair and check your grounding. Replace it if it seems worn or incomplete; check that it reaches the center of the planet; bring it into present time. Find the center of your head and take a few minutes to gather yourself together. When we do energy work like this, we're claiming back part of our life, part of our own energy that was ousted by Other People's Energy.

You could visualize your havingness levels on an old mercury thermometer with increments from zero to 100. Or you could use a yardstick or tape measure or any other measuring device. You don't really have to see it – you could just postulate that it's there or you could consult your knowingness, your intuition. What number does it give you? Or you might hear a number being said to you.

Whichever scale you're using, just nudge the havingness up a little way. Pushing it up far doesn't work very well as it tends to fall back to its first position. That's because one's whole being needs to get used to the higher level and that might take a minute, a week, or months! So first get an idea of where it is and then nudge it up. Let's say we're looking at our havingness for fine quality dining. Pictures might pop up like witches or ghosts at some amusement park ride.

"Noooo! Too expensive!"

"You're too fat already! Heh heh!"

Maybe cost pictures will waggle dollar signs at you. "You stick to junk food! Junk is your level! Ha!"

Just let such stuff go by without reacting to it. Ground it off. Keep your focus on the havingness gauge and where you want to set it for now. Tomorrow or next week you can nudge it up some more. Don't fight or get stuck in resistance. Resistance is Indeed Futile! For instance, if you're working on your health havingness, don't start arguments in your head, telling your doctor what for. Just calmly raise that gauge again, and the next day, check on it. If it slid down, raise it again. Do this as often as it takes to get your fine food or good health havingness remaining as high as you want it. Allow yourself to feel the increased certainty that comes with higher havingness.

Raising your havingness for something may have repercussions in your "space" – your body and energy field. Something has set that havingness where it is, and that something might not like it being changed. For example, if you have low havingness for good health:

- Perhaps your doctor has given you six months to live and flatly disbelieves that you might live for twelve months. Her authority looms over you, pressuring you to lower your good health havingness to fit her prediction.

- Perhaps you're 59 and your parents both died in their 60s and you assume you're genetically programmed to also die then. Science has decreed it! Who are you to defy scientific fact?

Our Western culture is unbalanced, it's so heavily rational. Proof! Where's the proof? Where are the scientific studies? We're taught to disbelieve anything that doesn't come with hundreds of double-blind placebo-controlled studies. That mitigates against us trusting our intuition.

That's "just your imagination".

"Hearing voices" is insanity!

If you "see things", you should be locked up or at least visit an eye doctor.

So be stubborn and keep your focus on your own bits of information. OPE is foreign to our own energy flow, intruding, tending to override what our own energy naturally wants to do. Becoming ourselves involves discarding OPE and claiming our own energy, owning it, giving it free run of our energy channels.

We don't need to allow other people to set our havingness levels. We can drain off that intrusive energy, drop it down the grounding cord, and replace it with our own creative energy complete with high havingness.

Memorandum

✓ Consider getting tests done to provide you with a picture of your health status;

✓ It's important to find out if your body can detoxify efficiently;

✓ Testing for vitamin and mineral deficiencies will tell you what foods to include in your diet or exclude from it and what supplements you might need to take;

✓ PEMF is a simple machine to use and gives you a myriad health benefits.

Chapter 8: Hyperthermia in Germany

My plane landed at the Frankfurt airport on a sunny Sunday in early July, 2014, and I was met by an Arcadia staff person I'll call Hans. He was cheerful and fatherly and made me feel well-looked-after. It was a two-hour drive to Bad Emstal and a beautiful one. I had to dig down to my memories of England at ages 10 to 12 to find anything as green as this German landscape. We passed through several villages and what struck me most, aside from the bright flowers and greenery, was the solidity of the houses: two-stories, brick, or with half-timbering that made me feel I was about to meet Shakespeare.

The name "Bad Emstal" might sound a bit alarming to an English speaker but "Bad" means "Spa". Germans put their adjectives after their nouns. We were heading for the village called Emstal Spa along some side roads and when we arrived, there was the spa, part of the Arcadia complex. Being Sunday, the place was still and peaceful, the other resident patients not here yet or perhaps napping in their rooms. Two women met us, speaking German and exuding hospitality. They turned out to be cleaning women who were getting the place ready for Monday's new patients.

They showed me up to my room and Hans brought my baggage. Then he went home to his family and one of the women, I'll call her Bridgitt, showed me where clean linen was kept and which other rooms were still empty or now occupied. There were five completed rooms and more still under construction. It was still transition time between the clinic's previous location in Kassel, and this new one that was still being built and equipped. After I'd put my clothing away and inspected the wild greenery outside the glass doors in my outside wall, and the as-yet-unbuilt verandah, I went downstairs and through the entry area, taking my walking stick. Stacks of wood, carpentry tools, and electrician-looking things decorated the wide staircase area, bright daylight bathing it all through the glass walls and windows both sides.

From down the driveway, looking back at the buildings, I saw that two existing village houses had been connected by a new area containing the wide stairs from the left house to the right one, each three levels counting the basements. There was a path winding around the left side of this building complex so I followed it, flowering bushes brushing me on each side, and came to another building further left with a large bricked area in front of it. It was closed but through the glass doors I could see a big circular lobby with a fountain. I later learned that it was spa water, excellent for health improvement. To the left of it was the entrance to the Spa itself and to the right, a dining room with a long verandah full of tables and chairs. I could see part of a buffet on the right, empty and gleaming spic and span for Monday's customers who would include all us cancer patients as well as local spa visitors.

Soon I felt overwhelmed and returned to my room to lie down. I was in Bach's country! Schubert's country, the country of Beethoven, Mozart, Strauss, Brahms, Wagner, Schumann, Liszt, and Haydn. How did this small country produce so many top-quality musicians for so long? Handel's country too though he moved to London and became the court musician there. My consciousness flooded with phrases and fragments from all these composers, many of whose songs, sonatas or concertos I'd learned and played years ago. I fell asleep with Bach's second Brandenburg Concerto pounding in my heart.

The name *Arcadia* comes from a central mountainous area of Greece that in ancient times was populated by rural people whose lifestyle was unmarred by conquering armies or dictatorial invaders. The mountains protected them. It was Pan's country, the god of woods, shepherds, flocks of sheep and rustic music. Think of how panpipes sound – expressive of the breeze, of rural peace, and lots of space. The name *Arcadia* has often been used to symbolize an innocent and rural life, a "back to basics" idea.

Monday morning breakfast was a sociable affair. I met Solweig from Sweden and Jimmie from Texas and Dr. Sebastian* who arrived on his electric bicycle. The buffet for us cancer patients offered a hot main dish, a salad bar, and side items like sauerkraut and pickles and yogurt, all good for the gut, as well as toast on the assumption that we knew not to overindulge in carbohydrates. Dr. Sebastian answered questions and I learned that he didn't mind us having a morning cup of coffee. Just one cup per day wasn't harmful in his view.

Local Hyperthermia

We each received a printed schedule for the day. First thing Monday, I had an hour with Dr. Saupe, the medical director, who would direct my care. He is a tall, slim man with

---

* Not his real name

a ready smile and time to talk to you. His medical specialty is oncology and he carries a lot of responsibility running the clinic. He took a prick of my blood and we looked at it in his dark field microscope. The red cells were a bit less clumped than I'd seen them before (p. 141), though on the slide, they moved briskly for just six or seven minutes rather than the 30 or 40 minutes healthier cells could have done.

"Dr. Saupe, I have an important question."

"Call me Dr. Henning, Jen. We use first names around here. What's your question?"

"Is dark chocolate OK for a cancer patient?"

He laughed, his blue eyes twinkling. "Yes, if it's 70% or higher, that's fine. And cacao is a superfood, packed with nutrition."

That made my day. I thanked him for his time and went downstairs for my first treatment, local hyperthermia. Though it raised my temperature to 39^{0}C (102.2^{0}F), it was a restful treatment. Using electromagnetic energy at 13 megahertz frequency, it overheats the cancer cells and speeds their death but barely affects normal cells because they absorb less energy and warm up too minimally to be damaged. It also stimulates white blood cells into more police action.

For an hour or so I lay on the bed, torso covered by the special heating pad and with two IV drips into a vein: one giving bicarbonate of soda for body alkalinity and the other giving Artesunate (a form of Artemisia annua, Chinese wormwood, for stimulating cancer cell apoptosis). Another effect of local hyperthermia is stimulation of the body cells' mitochondria. These are tiny structures in every cell that make that cell's energy. That's how the body has energy, from each cell creating it.

Local hyperthermia also works on the gut. When I started to sit up afterwards, a strange movement happened in my belly. It lasted just four or five seconds. Neither before nor since have I felt anything like it. It felt like a creature crawling out of its burrow after a long hibernation. I hoped it was my intestinal white cells waking up after years of being suppressed, exhausted, shut down, and now starting to pursue pathogens. After that I slept till dinner time but "supper" at Arcadia was a light meal. I started to bring small amounts of food to our upstairs refrigerator in case of late night hunger. I've been a night owl for many years but here I had to be up and out by 8am for breakfast and ready for treatments at 9am. I used my trusty iPhone alarm.

Artesunate for Tumors

For tumorous cancers, Artesunate gives a double benefit.

- As tumors grow, they pull iron from the body and this creates anemia. An Artesunate treatment is therefore preceded by an iron infusion. Now the tumors are very full of iron so when the Artesunate enters them, a lot of free radicals are released that do what they do anywhere: damage tissue. This breaks up the tumor by destroying its cells.

- Artesunate also reduces the formation of blood vessels supplying tumor cells, making metastasis less likely.

Artesunate is on the World Health Organization's list of Essential and Important Medicines. It is derived from Chinese mugwort (Artesunate annua)

---Adapted from Arcadia's webpage on Artesunate Infusions.

The next day was local hyperthermia again, with IV vitamin C this time and oxygen inhalation, and an EKG in preparation for the following day's full body hyperthermia. There was also a massage from one of the nurses during which I fell asleep. Wiped out, I went up to my room and slept for eight hours, missing dinner. Then I stayed up all night, on my Mac laptop, reading about cancer and treatments and the recent news and sending emails to friends.

Full Body Hyperthermia

This was a dramatic treatment indeed. On this first time, they made it a half hour shorter, down to one hour, as I was feeling nauseous and stressed from hurrying to breakfast and back for this treatment.

My nurse was Hang (pronounced Haang), a friendly and cheerful woman whose parents had escaped from Vietnam and she was born in Laos but mostly grew up in Germany. She was also fluent in English and Vietnamese. I have enormous admiration for multi-lingual people. She went about making me comfortable while securing all the necessary attachments to some part of me or other:

- A device to the left earlobe to monitor my pulse rate;
- A thermometer in the rectum to monitor body core temperature;
- An oxygen cannula in my nostrils;
- An IV line to a vein in my right arm that would deliver a high dose of vitamin C.

I lay on my back and when everything was in place and I stopped wriggling, she closed the curved lid over me and clamped it onto the frame of the sling arrangement I lay on. That gave me a slight trapped feeling but I grounded it off and filled myself up with my best orange-gold healing energy.

"Could you move that monitor to where I can see it, Hang?"

She laughed. "No, there are no wheels. I take good care of you Jenny. I watch the monitor for you. It shows me your temperature rising."

She draped a shiny camping blanket over the top of the curved lid.

"This will reflect lid heat back to you." She tucked it close under my chin so I was cocooned inside this big device and totally in her care. I relaxed and decided to enjoy this treatment. Soon I felt the warmth increasing and I began to sweat. Hang was right there with a towel to mop my face and head and offer me sips of water through a straw. My temperature increased slowly and steadily and sweat poured off my whole body.

"This is good detox, Jen. Lots of toxins coming out in that sweat."

She allowed my temperature to reach 40^0 centigrade (104^0 Fahrenheit), staying with me, mopping, offering water and chatting some. At one point I asked if she could lower the temperature a bit.

"Which part of you feels too hot?"

"My legs. They feel burning hot."

Hang moved to the other end of the hyperthermia device and turned a knob.

"You tell me when your legs feel more comfortable."

Soon they did and I finished the treatment feeling hot but safe. When the hour was up, Hang removed the IV line, oxygen tube, rectal thermometer and ear lobe pulse monitor and helped me out to a bed a few feet away made up with fresh thick cotton sheets. She wrapped me up and I lay there for a while cooling down. She moved around re-arranging things and putting a fresh sheet in the device.

"I'll get your lunch now Jen. You stay there till I get back."

I dozed off and soon she was back. I sat in the same room, wrapped in the sheet, and ate off my lap. Another delicious anti-cancer meal.

Arcadia had a downstairs with a PEMF machine that anyone could use. I started a habit of going down there after dinner each night. All the staff was gone home and I turned on the corridor light to see my way and then the room light. I loved the quiet ambience. For more on PEMF, see pp. 141-142.

(Continued on p. 155)

> Give me a chance to create a fever and I will cure any disease.
>
> ---Parmenides, Greek physician and philosopher, 540 to 480 B.C.

More About Hyperthermia

Hyperthermia for cancer was developed in the 1930s by Baron Manfred von Ardenne in Germany. It was part of his "three-point cancer treatment" along with oxygen and high-dose vitamin C, 30 grams or more.

Fever is not an illness. It's the body's reaction to a toxic invasion and should usually be allowed to run its course. The increased heat eventually kills invading bacteria while leaving healthy body cells unaffected. Of course a feverish person should be well-cared for with extra water to drink and their body temperature monitored.

The hyperthermia-elevated temperature has the same effect as a natural fever, signaling the immune system that something is wrong, that the white cells must wake up and chase down the invaders. And as they do this, they detect cancer cells and disable them for later excretion.

Because hyperthermia treatments are done along with IV vitamin C, the detoxification is greatly increased. When we take a vitamin C tablet, it acts as an antioxidant. But when we receive 30 grams or more directly into the blood, bypassing the digestive system, it acts as an oxidant, an oxidizer, and attaches itself to other molecules.

Vitamin C molecules are the same size as those of glucose and when a large number of vitamin C molecules are in the body, cancer cells pull them in; they go in through the "glucose tunnel", i.e. deceptively using the insulin receptors on the cell's membrane.

Cancer cells have many extra insulin receptors on their membranes, enabling them to gobble up much more of whatever glucose is available and mistakenly gobble up more vitamin C. The vitamin C then interacts with other things in the cells, producing hydrogen peroxide. As this process continues, hydrogen peroxide builds up until it breaks the cancer cell, killing it. Healthy cells are unaffected.

The use of oxygen during hyperthermia is the third item in this 3-point treatment. Cancer develops only when the body cells are deficient in oxygen and during hyperthermia, with cancer cells open for glucose but instead receiving vitamin C, they also receive extra oxygen. Oxygen is unwelcome since cancer cells have abandoned it in favor of fermenting glucose for their energy. It encourages the cell to revert to normal use of oxygen, becoming non-cancerous.

Treatments and Events

Each evening, using the Mac laptop, I made notes about that day's events. The following is from those notes. They don't cover every daily detail but I hope they give a picture of life and treatments at Arcadia.

Thursday July 3

Had a session with Dr. Christian Büttner, a Psycho-oncologist. Like Dr. Saupe, he's a tall, capable man with a calm demeanour. He said, "Be in your bones where blood is made." He also said, "Put a crystal wall around your aura for protection." I was amazed that he seemed to know about energy work. And he knew that I knew and would understand him.

"Ground yourself more. After you've been sociable and allowed people into your space, be alone and push them out. Own your space."

It was true that I was not staying well enough grounded here – I was in ongoing over-stimulation what with the familiar-but-unknown German language, the new people and surroundings, and the powerful treatments, and I was stretching to get my understanding around those things, forgetting to maintain and protect my space. I began to like this man. Then he said,

"Your mother game is over so move on." My older son, who has schizophrenia, was recently in hospital to have his intestines cleared; they were entirely blocked. The staff where he lived were not caring for him well enough. I feel that my mothering days are not over with him. So I didn't agree with Dr. Büttner. (Later, my younger son Dmitri and I found Chris a better residence .)

"Your boys are men now. It's time for you to stop worrying about them."

This upset me and I got a bit teary. I went up to my room and slept an hour or so and then was late to lunch. One of the Spa staff came to me in the dining room saying, "The doctor is waiting for you. They're looking for you." I grew angry and a little later argued with one of the nurses.

(It wasn't her fault; I was "lit up" as they say in my energy world: I had "grief pictures" lit up about my motherhood and my son who can't work and support himself yet is very intelligent and talented in music and drawing. Dr. Büttner had put me into a "growth period" – I was processing energy and not fully present to those around me. Of course, he was doing his job and he'd done it deftly too; I had to admire that.)

Local hyperthermia that afternoon. We had red wine at dinner, another pleasant exception like the one morning cup of coffee to the "no-no"s of an anti-cancer diet.

Friday July 4

We have a new version of the schedule with the treatment names in English. I like it! Talked for over an hour with Dr. Saupe about many topics; I find him very easy to be with. I asked him,

"Dr. Henning, what do you think about the pleomorphic microbe theory of cancer causation?"

"I don't subscribe to it, Jen."

"Even though Royal Rife and many others have seen those microbes inside cancer cells and seen them moving around, alive?"

"Yes. I don't deny that such microbes are present in cancer cells but their presence does not prove any causative connection to the disease. They might be a result of cancer rather than a cause. There are other microbes in there too."

"So what would you say is the main cause of cancer?"

"I'm not convinced there is any 'main cause'. I think there are many contributing causes that converge at some point and by their preponderance tip the body into a cancerous state; convert some of the body cells to anaerobic fermentation of sugar for their energy rather than use of oxygen."

"OK. So lack of oxygen would be one of those contributing causes."

"Yes. The lack of oxygen eventually forces some body cells to resort to sugar metabolism. That's a survival mechanism. Those cells are struggling to stay alive, and with plenty of glucose available, they become anaerobic, giving up on trying to obtain enough oxygen." (For more on cancer causes, see Chapter 10.)

Dr. Saupe did a stress test, having me sit still for five minutes with an electrode around each wrist. I scored 54%, a pretty good score in the middle range of parasympathetic stress. Maybe he had heard about my session with Dr. Büttner and my tendency to lateness and wanted to see if I was still upset. I wasn't.

He arranged for an ultrasound treatment next Friday to check that all my abdominal organs are structurally normal.

Later I had local hyperthermia with IV Artemisia and then slept for two hours. These treatments are powerful! PEMF after dinner.

Saturday July 5

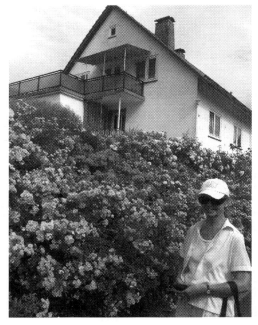

Solweig on our walk in beautiful Bad Emstal.

---Photo by Jen Kimberley

Woke at 4:30am and tossed around; Got up at 5:30 and snacked on some sheep cheese and dried beef. How excellent that we have this large refrigerator upstairs near our private rooms. After breakfast, Solweig and I went for a walk around the village, admiring the flowers, the tidy front yards, the old brick buildings that looked so clean. We met up with Jimmie and walked together. I took photos. The village seemed to have no downtown, not even any shops. Eventually we came upon one here and one there; no billboards, no big signs, just a doorway that opened into a small grocery shop or newspaper shop. Hardly any people in the streets. I slept from 4pm to 7:30pm and then was too wide awake to sleep the rest of the night. I downloaded Bad Emstal photos to the Mac, read some news and emails, read a good novel, and got clothes and snacks ready for Sunday's field trip.

Sunday July 6

Hans, who had picked me up at the Frankfurt airport, drove us to a local sort-of-castle for a morning field trip. We were Solweig, Jimmie, me and another man, a Swedish cancer patient whom I didn't get to know. The fifth patient was more severely ill and stayed a lot in her room. The sort-of-castle was in Kassel and was built over the years of 1700 to 1717 by a man with a huge ego. To get there we drove up a high hill and once there, we climbed up many steps, and at the top was an enormous statue of the builder as Hercules.

He stood overlooking the beautiful valley and the view of Kassel spread out for his inspection. A wide road with wide areas of greenery along each side ran directly from far below the foot of this statue into Kassel and I couldn't help but picture this ruler stepping down from his giant pedestal and striding imperiously along the wide road to investigate some wrongdoing he'd spied among his serfs. The buildings around his statue were covered in scaffolding and staff told us that it was permanently there because the original bricks were crumbling and needed ongoing repairs. I call it a sort-of-castle because it didn't have turrets or a moat and drawbridge; it wasn't war-oriented. But it was built on the sort of site that castles tend to occupy: high up for detecting enemy troops in the distance.

After lunch, I went with Jimmie to a village "Project", a café serving coffee and wine. It was owned and run by a woman using inherited money, she told us, and her targeted customers were musicians and homeless people; others were welcome too. She serves inexpensive meals to the homeless though I don't think there are many of them in Bad Emstal.

Jimmie and I settled in and ordered coffee. Jimmie was a gentleman with courteous manners. In a sense, he looked after me, opening the door, pulling out a chair for me, waiting for me if I lagged behind as we walked around Bad Emstal. In my view, it's a great pity that men have largely been persuaded out of that gentlemanly behavior to women. Since I've used the walking stick, I've particularly noticed the change and have been almost knocked down sometimes by men barging in front of me or letting a door slam in my face. On the other side of the coin, I especially appreciate it when a man does show courtesy.

A pianist was accompanying a woman who played her guitar and sang Big Band songs. At the table next to us, a banjo player was waiting to play. If I'd had my fiddle and no finger arthritis I would have got in line too and played German classical tunes from memory such as Beethoven's *Adelaide* or Schubert's *The Trout*. I bet an accompanist would have appeared too.

Four men -- a singer, sax player and two guitarists -- started singing some Beatles songs, using recorded drums, but I was falling asleep now. No sleep last night and treatments tomorrow at 9:30am. The staff had loosened my schedule a bit because I couldn't hurry enough (though I was always trying to hurry). I slept 4pm to 1:30am.

Monday July 7

Up in the wee hours, I decided to go downstairs for a PEMF treatment and found Jimmie's email address under my door. After PEMF, I saw the taxi outside and realized Jimmie was leaving so we had our last conversation and a hug in the pre-dawn. Back to my Mac and good novel. After breakfast, it was local hyperthermia with IV Artemisia and this time, Dr. Sebastian inserted the needle. The nurses have had trouble with my veins ever since I arrived; Dr. Sebastian said they were weakened by the leukemia pills.

Tuesday July 8

Had a Tibetan Bowl treatment today. That's instead of a massage as the massage nurse became ill around my second day here and will be out sick the rest of my time. For the Tibetan Bowls, I lay on the massage table while one of the nurses used six or eight bowls of different sizes and pitches, allowing the sound to almost fade before tapping the next one. The vibrations are beautiful in their subtle layers of sound, especially when two reverberate together, and they floated me into an almost-trance state. As the last tone faded, the ambient quietness wrapped around me – there is no traffic noise at Arcadia. Also had full body hyperthermia. Hang never minds if I'm sleepy; it goes with the treatment.

Wednesday July 9

Had a food allergy test a week ago and today Dr. Sebastian went over the results with me. Thankfully, most foods are in Group One, the OK list, but there are three other lists containing most of my favorite foods.

- Group Two: avocado, pineapple, hazelnuts and green beans to be eaten only every three or four days.

- Group Three: Eggs and garlic eliminated for at least two months;

- Group Four: All nuts and seeds except sesame eliminated for at least three months; also all milk from any motherly creature God ever thought of making. That's because they all contain Casein.

"No dairy of any sort for at least six months!" said Dr. Sebastian.

So no more midnight sheep cheese. Surprisingly, I'm not allergic to gluten or lactose, two common allergens.

Local hyperthermia today with IV vitamin C and oxygen. Dr. Sebastian got the needle in again. At dinner, talked to Solweig about her book on cancer. It's published in Swedish so I can't read it but she emailed me the cover. We sipped our red wine and exchanged lots of information since I was writing this Saga too. Sent an email to Jimmie – missing his warm presence.

Thursday July 10

After full body hyperthermia I crashed and slept 4pm to 9:30, missing dinner. Solweig put some dinner for me in the fridge and a note under my door.

Friday July 11

Slept 2am to 6:30. Had abdominal ultrasound from a doctor who works with both local people and us resident cancer patients. He found normality everywhere except on the right kidney where there was a small cyst, but he said it's rather common and nothing to worry about. In my hour with Dr. Henning I suggested that all our rooms have a lamp for reading. During lunch, someone put a floor lamp in my room! This is a very caring place; I feel it in the atmosphere every day. Dr. Henning put a needle in my left hand for an oxygen treatment and all seems well.

Weekend of July 12-13

On Saturday, Solweig and I had breakfast together and walked in the big village park. Later, she returned to Sweden. We exchanged emails until her death.*****

On Sunday, I sat alone in the dining room reading another good novel and sipping coffee with coconut milk. Members of a small women's choir assembled and I listened to them rehearsing. Then I walked in the park, missing Solweig and Jimmie. Some new people arrived and I talked to a couple from Singapore.

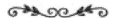

I was at Arcadia until July 23. In one of my hours with Dr. Saupe, he told me about his adventures running a cancer clinic in Sweden. It was highly successful with people

---

* Solweig died of her cancer in 2017 after home care from doctors, nurses, and a dietitian. Her sons cared for her and were present to the end. As I write this in 2019, I'm still sad to have lost her.

applying from many countries, having read about it in newspaper coverage. He then had to close it down. I later wrote an account of it that he approved and I'll post it at jenkimberley.com.

There were more treatments and tests done for me at Arcadia than are mentioned in the diary notes:

- Ozone to clean the blood;

- A stool test to check on how well I was digesting foods;

- IV Dichloroacetate (DCA) which stimulates the subdued mitochondria in cancer cells, causing them to signal their cancer cell to commit apoptosis;

- A Heparin shot to thin the blood against a high platelet count;

- Oral supplements such as proteolytic enzymes, curcumin, vitamin D, selenium, zeolite powder, and Quercetin.

On my last treatment day I had full body hyperthermia and chatted with Hang.

"What will you do when you go home, Jen?"

"Good question, Hang. I don't know. I'm staying with a friend in Denver and we used to go dancing a lot. Now I stay home and she goes dancing."

"I wish I could dance. I want to take lessons."

I grinned up at her from under the shiny blanket over the machine's cover. "I'll show you today if you like. I'll try not to fall over."

She laughed and I saw her eyes flash with pleasure at the idea. After the treatment was finished and I was dressed, I took her hand.

"Let's do a Country Two-Step. I'll sing the music."

We went out the door to the wide corridor. It was the basement level and the stairs were on our left. The rest of the corridor was lined both sides with offices and treatment rooms and ran to a glass exit door at the far end. This was the corridor I walked along each night to the PEMF room, last on the left. I started singing a country song from the 1980s and took Hang into the ballroom position with me as the man. I'm not a dance teacher and don't know men's parts but for a basic two-step I figured I could manage.

"Slow – slow – quick quick; Slow – slow – quick quick." I steered her backwards as the female does it and led her in the steps. She caught on quickly and we danced the length of the corridor and back, me bellowing the song with joy, happy to be dancing after two years of inability for it, and Hang laughing.

Some		Bro-	ken	hearts	never	mend;	
S	S	Q - Q	S	S	Q - Q	S	S
---	Some	mem	-ories	ne----	----ver	end;	
Q - Q	S	S	Q - Q	S	S	Q - Q	S

"Some tears will never dry, And my love for you will never die."*

Then I turned both of us together on some of the "slow – slows". When she got that I started to spin her gently on some of the "fast fasts" and at first she was startled but soon got it. She had a natural ability for dancing. People appeared in the doorways laughing with amazement. Dr. Henning was at the bottom of the stairs when we danced back again to that end of the corridor, clapping and laughing.

The amazing thing for me was that I didn't stumble or fall. Hang didn't prop me up but just having that dance partner hold gave me a sense of "Up". I was very excited to think I might be able to get back to dancing after all.

I left Arcadia with six syringes of Heparin and instructions to give them to myself, one each day. I did that. I had done it previously too, in Arizona, using Lovenox, a form of Heparin. They reduce platelet numbers. CML pushes the platelets up and the red cells down but sometimes it just pushes the white cell count up (by making lots of dysfunctional white cells) and leaves the others normal. Lots of monitoring called for.

On my last day Hans drove me to the Frankfurt airport. People came out to say goodbye and share hugs: tall, kind Elof from Norway, who didn't mind that I disagreed with his view of the EU; frail Lin from Singapore (I hugged him very carefully); friendly, sensible Marie from France; Alexie and Benita from Denmark. It's amazing what warm friendships can develop in a short time between cancer patients. We understand each

---

* "Some Broken Hearts Never Mend", written by American song writer Wayland Holyfield, recorded by country music artist Don Williams, released in 1977 in his album, *Visions*. https://www.youtube.com/watch?v=Fi0vmnxM3ao

other's situation and want the best for each other, yet know that it might not be achieved. I felt that I could stay at Arcadia indefinitely.

Heartfelt thanks to Dr. Henning Saupe for his kindness and patience with me and for his many answers to questions and his interview about the clinic in Sweden. Heartfelt thanks also to Dr. Sebastian for his kind and attentive medical care and answers about diet; and to Dr. Büttner for putting me into a growth period so expertly. How could we grow spiritually without growth periods?! I could not have been better cared for anywhere in the world than I was at Arcadia Klinik. (Narrative continues on p. 167)

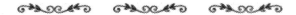

Memorandum

✓ Hyperthermia is an induced fever that tells your immune system you are not well. It thus stimulates your white blood cells to go after any invaders and that would include cancer cells.

✓ Hyperthermia is potentiated by being done concurrently with IV vitamin C and oxygen. Since body cells turn cancerous when oxygen is lacking, an extra supply of it helps them revert to normal aerobic functioning. The vitamin C at that high IV dose is an oxidizer and zaps pathogens.

✓ Quality time with your cancer doctor can be a blessing that allows you to get answers and calm any frustration and anxiety you may have.

✓ There are many benign treatments for cancer; we have choices other than chemo, surgery or radiation.

✓

✓

✓

Chapter 9: Offsetting Chemo Harm

Iinclude this chapter because most cancers involve tumors although my leukemia doesn't. The information here is thus not based on my own experience but drawn from what I have read online and in books and have heard from doctors and from cancer patients who do have tumors.

Tumors Are Not Cancer

It's important to get clear on the difference between tumors and Cancer itself. Tumorous cancers, the majority of cancers, are more alarming and distressing than my invisible blood cancer, just because they feature growths that have no business being on or in your body, and associated pain. With ongoing pain it would be very understandable if a person agreed quickly to surgery to remove the growth, or if they allowed their doctor to hurry them into chemotherapy. Many people start chemo thinking that it will kill the cancer and that although they might feel sick for a while and lose their hair, in the long run they'll recover, their hair will grow back, and they'll be finished with cancer. They'll be "in remission", and from the viewpoint of someone in pain and fear, "in remission" might sound as good as "cured".

There is a widespread tendency for tumors to be spoken of as if they are the cancer, so that disposing of tumors equals disposing of cancer. It is common to hear talk of "cancer cells" meaning "tumor cells".

Tumors are not the cancer. They are a **symptom** of cancer and the cancer itself is systemic – that's why it "returns". It never went away because treatments typically do not target the cancerous **stem cells** that proliferate tumor cells; they target the tumor cells, the daughter cells created by the cancerous stem cells. That's why "in remission" does not mean "cured". The cancer itself is established, entrenched, in the body, and has been for months or years before any medical test has been able to pick up on it. At diagnosis time, it's cruising, powered by factors such as sugary artificial food, insufficient body movement (i.e. lack of oxygen), polluted air, contaminated tap water, chemicals leached from clothing, and poisons in personal care products and household furnishings. Not to mention negative emotions: pessimism as to outcome, anger at the doctor, the cancer, the treatment, the healthcare system, the world. If these influences are not removed, the cancer continues thriving after conventional treatments, strengthens, and produces new tumors. Actually, tumors are body tissue enclosing cancerous tissue – the body trying to contain this illness. Typically the cancer is stronger and more aggressive when it "returns" because it has been growing while the patient was "in remission".

Disposing of the environmental influences is our job as cancer patients because they are in our personal and home surroundings where we have some control. Improving our diet is also our job; and grounding off negative emotions. To divest ourselves of cancer we must lighten the mood, nourish and detoxify the body, and clean up our surroundings as much as we can. If our cancer is ever to be cured, it's our immune system that will do it. But it needs our help.

Be the Captain of Your Ship

The idea of your food or home promoting your cancer might seem baffling or shocking but if you look closer, it's comforting and encouraging. It gives you power. These are things you have control over. You are not some disabled boat being thrown around in rough seas – your body is that boat and you, the person living in the body, are the ship's captain. You can organize activity on board to bail seawater out, block leaks, toss away broken and unneeded items, and stabilize important items; (that is, remove toxins, take supplements, toss away processed "food", and form new healthier habits). You can employ your doctor as one of your sailors: let him or her attend to the cancer symptom while you attend to the cancer itself, navigating your ship into safe waters.

You probably have other crew members ready to work: maybe a chef, a cabin steward, or some sturdy deck hands. If you work with a supportive team, your chances of success are much higher, as you won't be so susceptible to low moods or giving up.

If you opt for conventional treatment, you can prepare for it, defend yourself against its potential destruction, and compensate for any losses it will cause. The more you know about your upcoming treatment, the better you can prepare for it. That is information you can obtain if you do your reading and ask questions of your doctor. Take a notebook and pen and make clear notes.

Ten Questions to Ask Your Doctor

1. **What exactly is my diagnosis?**

Get the exact name and stage; then get a second opinion. You could get a third opinion if you want the extra reassurance as to accuracy. Sometimes people are given a cancer diagnosis when they actually have some other condition. If you are told you have a "pre-cancerous" lesion, this is not a cancer diagnosis. It refers to a growth that might turn out to be a tumor but might not. Some doctors might urge you to have it removed surgically right away, just "in case" it becomes malignant. However, if it is cancer, it's already malignant, and if it isn't, a ship's captain can direct changes in diet and lifestyle to greatly reduce any chance of future malignancy.

2. **Do I have a fast-growing cancer or slow?**

If it's fast-growing, you still have time to learn and think and decide. Don't let anyone frighten you into a bad decision. If it's slow-growing, you can better combat any rushing or sense of panic.

3. **What drugs will you treat me with?**

There will probably be several. Write down their names for research and future reference.

4. **Might I need other drugs as well, along the way?**

Drugs may be given to reduce the side effects of other drugs or to address problems that might come up unexpectedly.

5. **What are the short-term side effects of those drugs?**

Don't accept a referral to the paperwork that comes with each drug. It will likely be too obscure and printed in a tiny font that nobody can read without eyestrain. Ask your doctor to spell it out in plain English and take notes.

6. **What are the long-term side effects?**

Again, let the doctor spell it out, even if he or she is wanting to move on to the next patient. You deserve to be fully informed about whatever harm you will be susceptible to.

7. **Are any of these side effects life-threatening?**

There'll be the relatively minor side effects like nausea, loss of appetite, full-body discomfort 24/7, and hair loss. But these toxic drugs have major side effects that you deserve to be forewarned about. Examples are brain damage, liver, kidney and bladder damage, and new secondary cancers. There could even be "sudden death from cardiac arrest", as was the case with a new drug my conventional doctor offered to me.

8. **Will the drugs cure my cancer or just relieve the symptoms?**

The true answer is "relieve the symptoms". No chemo drug cures cancer. The doctor might talk about extending your life or enhancing its quality, but you might not agree that living a few weeks or months longer is a huge benefit; or that spending months feeling damaged and sick is much of a life-enhancement.

9. **I've heard that chemotherapy drugs make the cancer more aggressive. Is that true?**

Chemo drugs do in effect make the cancer more aggressive because they weaken your immune system and general health so you're less able to combat the cancer. They also enable some cancers to become resistant to the drugs and more strongly-based in the body. And with no teaching about how to strengthen your weakened immunity or how to remove carcinogens from your home or diet, you'll be allowing your cancer free rein to grow more fierce – unless, of course, you have appointed yourself captain of your ship and will be seeing to the cancer while the doctor is seeing to the symptom.

10. **What would be the best anti-cancer diet to adopt?**

This is an exploratory question to see if the doctor has any awareness of good nutrition or of sugary junk foods feeding cancer. Does the office have a bowl of free wrapped candies for patients? As mentioned earlier in this Saga (p.50). I could find no anti-cancer menu in the big hospital binder they gave me to order dinner from. It contained a menu for diabetics, one for people sensitive to gluten, one for those wanting to keep their weight down, and many others, but none for patients wanting to discourage cancer. If your doctor displays ignorance of nutrition, there'll be no changing his or her mind. But you can set about seeing to your own nutrition improvement.

> Inaction breeds doubt and fear. Action breeds confidence and courage. If you want to conquer fear, do not sit home and think about it. Go out and get busy.
>
> ---Dale Carnegie

Theoretically, there are two successful approaches to treating cancer:

1. Kill the cancer cells while boosting the immune system to cope better;

2. Revert the cancer cells to normal use of oxygen.

By going with chemo you're choosing option 1, and as your ship's captain, improving your health and strengthening your immunity will greatly increase the chances of chemo success.

Option 2 is not typically offered by conventional doctors. You would need to either look for an alternative cancer clinic or choose a protocol you could do at home on your own and with appropriate testing, you could probably customize any of the do-it-yourself protocols. (See Chapter 10 for more on protocols.)

Some Possible Pre-Chemo Measures

If you will be having repeated intravenous treatments, your doctor may suggest having **a device inserted, such as a port**, to avoid your having to be pricked each time. Page 43 has a picture of my port and description of how it worked. That would be a great blessing given how much discomfort is usually unavoidable when having chemo.

Your doctor may also suggest **a dental visit** to make sure you have no infection in your mouth, no gum disease or incipient cavities. Chemo will decimate your immune system, reducing its ability to deal with infection.

If your doctor does not suggest a dental visit, you could do it anyway. Find a biologic dentist; they consider the health of the whole body when putting any given dental material in a person's mouth.

- **Health Risks of Mercury**

    You might want to read up about metal in the mouth. Dental amalgam is about half mercury and half a metal alloy. Mercury is one of the most poisonous substances on earth, along with the botulinum toxin, cyanide, mustard gas and a few others. Whenever we put hot drinks or food in our mouth – typically many times each day – the mercury in fillings gives off tiny amounts of vapor which enter our sinuses and nasal cavities. Mercury in the body can lead to many health problems. If you can find a biologic dentist, consider having metal amalgam fillings replaced with safe ceramic fillings. Biologic dentists use protective measures when they drill out amalgam. For example, they place a "dam" in the mouth to prevent mercury particles from being swallowed and masks on everyone's faces, including their own, to prevent breathing of mercury fumes.

- **Health Risks of Fluoride**

  Biologic dentists do not use or recommend fluoride. Applied topically in toothpaste it can be beneficial but ingesting it as a medication in public water supplies has not been shown to confer any dental benefits. The EU banned it years ago. Research has also been showing that fluoride disrupts the body's endocrine system. A huge array of health problems can result from this; examples are arthritis, thyroid dysfunction, decreased male fertility, increased lead absorption, and weakened bones leading to bone fractures and bone cancer. We can filter fluoride out of our water with a filtering jug or a filter that fits on the pipe bringing water to the house.

In some cases, **medical tests** are recommended to check your body's ability to deal with the chemo onslaught. There'll be a rush of dead cancer cells to be excreted, along with the toxins they release upon being killed and any microbes that were living inside them, also now dead. Your liver and kidneys will be working hard to cope with all this so they need to be in reasonably good health. There may also be a cardiac test.

- **Captains**: Hulda Clark devised good kidney and liver cleanses, available online. And consider doing coffee enemas. See p. 62-63 for how they work and p. 63-64 to learn how fortunate we are in being able to buy stainless steel enema buckets. ☺

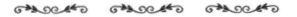

Memorandum

✓ Tumors are a symptom of cancer, not the cancer itself;

✓ Employ your doctor as a crew member in charge of treating the symptom while you attend to healing yourself of cancer;

✓ Ask your doctor lots of questions and take notes to get a clear picture of whatever treatment he or she plans for you;

✓ Do as much reading as you can to educate yourself about chemo or whichever treatment your doctor is recommending (radiation or surgery);

✓

✓

✓

Chapter 10: Devising a New Protocol

When I came back to Denver from Germany (September 2014), I had decided to return to my birth country, Australia, for a while. I had been homesick for years for the tuneful and varied birdsong, the gum trees with their fresh aroma, the fabulous surf beaches with their lifesaving clubs, and the sound of Aussie talk. So I moved to the Gold Coast area of Queensland where we used to have beach vacations in the September school holidays. I soon took a bus to the nearest beach called Long Beach and tried to walk across the dry sand to the water's edge, but of course I immediately fell. Dry sand shifts so easily and when my feet get tilted, turned sideways from being flat on flat ground, my fragile sense of "up" disappears. So I sat on the dry sand and watched the waves as I had in my teen years, unable now to run out with a glide and get rides, but very much enjoying the sights and sounds and sun, and the happiness of being on an Aussie beach again.

Living in Queensland, I went on to the Bill Henderson protocol fully (not partially as I had in Canada) and I became one of his coachees. I connected with a doctor, a short walk up the hill and into a small medical office, and saw her monthly. A petite woman in her 80s: high heels, long gray hair piled high haphazardly, pretty dresses. She was a conventional doctor but sweet-natured and had spent many years practicing in Alice Springs, dealing with sunstroke, snake bites and severe dehydration as well as occasional cancer. She gave me the full 20 minutes but we typically spent them with her listening in wonder at my alternative approaches to cancer. I wanted her opinions. But at the end of each visit, she humorously dismissed it all by saying, "Don't forget to take your Sprycel!" (the official leukemia pill). She had never encountered a leukemia patient who had lived longer than ten years from diagnosis.

During the two years I lived in Queensland, I started writing this book and stayed steady on the Bill Henderson protocol. I had a friend a few doors down and got to know my other neighbors, sharing a garden hose with Ruby next door for our flowers, and buying my vegetables from an organic stall in the nearby Farmers Market. We chatted some days when things weren't too busy. He uses permaculture – growing vegetables interspersed with native plants – and he told me how his non-organic neighbor sprayed the tomatoes seven times as they grew. How can we wash off pesticides that are incorporated into the vegetable's substance?

Then back in America in 2016 to be near my older son, I continued the Bill Henderson protocol but gradually lost confidence that it was being effective for me. It has been effective for a great many people but I'd had this leukemia for longer (15 years) than is typical when a person starts the protocol so perhaps it had become too strongly established in my system for "healing cancer gently" (wording that Bill Henderson used).

Something to keep in mind about cancer is that typically it tags along. First we develop other health problems, dealing with each one through drug store items or perhaps prescribed medications. Examples would be digestive problems, skin eruptions, headaches and joint pain. We get used to having these and continue our life activities until the big C diagnosis lands with a crash. That focuses our attention on health and hopefully we also start looking at how we've been living and eating. In my case, gas-and-constipation had been my long-term problem, resisting treatments by bentonite, montmorillonite clay, zeolite, takesumi, psyllium, and other such remedies, as well as an increase of water intake.

Uninvited Company

In 2017, to help with the gas-and-constipation problem, I started using Essiac. This is a herbal tea used by Nurse Rene Caisse (pronounced "Reen Case") in Canada back in the 1930s. She boiled it up in her kitchen each night and gave a dose to all the (many) people she found in her front room the next morning.* So I made Essiac one gallon at a time and stored it in the fridge for daily doses before breakfast. I used the eight-herb version. After ordering Caisse to close her clinic, the Canadian government obtained her four-herb recipe and has been selling it for years. But Caisse moved to Washington D.C. and worked with a doctor there to improve the formula by adding four more herbs. Originally, it was from an old Ojibwa Indian medicine man who gave it to a relative of one of Caisse's patients when she was still the head nurse at Toronto General Hospital.

---

* For the interesting story of Essiac, how it was used by Rene Caisse to cure cancer, and how others reacted, see **the blogs** Healing Cancer With Herbs, Part 1 and Part 2 on my website. http://www.jenkimberley.com

After two months, I was headed for Phoenix (to see a biologic dentist and a friend) and then Mexico (for a class). I would be gone about six weeks so I took a bag of Essiac powder with me. Staying in a Phoenix Airbnb, I made Essiac and took daily doses as usual. One day, after about a week, I was in the bathroom and suddenly had company. A long white worm appeared! It was about 20" long and a minute later, a second one appeared. I was particularly flabbergasted because two years previously, as a coachee of Bill Henderson, I'd had testing done for parasites. That doctor had found three microscopic parasites and Candida. I had promptly taken his prescribed remedies for those and then thought, Well, Thank you, Bill, for that good suggestion. That's fungus and parasites taken care of. -- Ha!

The following day in Phoenix, two more long worms appeared. On closer examination, I found that each was actually three worms twisted around each other. So perhaps the total was now 12. This went on for two more months with shorter worms starting to appear and by the end of that time (by then back in Illinois) they were about a quarter of an inch long. Although there were just about 20 very long ones, the quantity of worms anywhere from 20" to one inch was enormous and the quarter-inch worms were so numerous that I'd put the overall total at about a thousand.

How could so many creatures have lived in my gut without me knowing? By that time I'd been doing coffee enemas off and on (mostly on) for four years, removing much debris each time. And I'd been eating organic for five years. So I'd been providing luxury accommodation for the worm kingdom but did evicting its residents solve my gas-and-constipation problem? No. But read on.

Grateful to at least have my own gut to myself but still at a loss regarding cancer, I turned my attention back to the leukemia. (Continued on p. 179)

What Causes Cancer?

If the cause of a health problem is known, it can be targeted by treatments and thus removed. But when the cause is unknown, money pours into research projects, theories sprout up, and differing approaches to healing are devised. It's like the old Indian parable of the elephant:

> Several blind men are arguing over what the elephant is. "It's a big stone wall!" says the man at the elephant's side. "No, it's a fat tree branch!" says the man in front of the elephant. "Nonsense, it's a rope!" says the man behind it. "You're all wrong!" says the man squatting below the elephant. "It's a big heavy stone!" They each draw a conclusion based on whatever partial evidence they've found.

We all have some number of cancer cells forming all the time and a healthy immune system chases them down. Why do they build up to the point of a cancer diagnosis in some of us but not in others? There are four main theories as to cancer cause and here are short notes on them:

1. A Lifestyle Disease

This theory underlies this Saga because it's the one I've encountered most often in the ten years since I started reading about cancer and receiving treatments from alternative or integrative cancer doctors. It holds that cancer is the end result of a cascade of contributing causes -- lifestyle choices or life events -- where those causes build up to a tipping point. If support is given to them by a toxic diet and lifestyle, the immune system becomes overworked and may even go dormant or shut down. Cell division of existing cancerous cells thus meets with little or no opposition and the quantity of cancerous cells increases exponentially until a medical test is able to detect them.

2. A Genetic Disease

This is the favored theory among conventional doctors. For unknown reasons, DNA damage occurs in one or more stem cells which triggers uncontrolled cell division. The damaged daughter cells of these damaged stem cells become tumor cells (or dysfunctional blood cells in the case of blood cancers). They continue to divide and multiply, growing the tumors indefinitely or cluttering the blood to dangerous levels. The treatments with this theory are chemotherapy, surgery and radiation and symptom relief is known as "remission".

3. An Infectious Disease

This theory holds that cancer is caused by a pleomorphic microbe, i.e., an entity able to change its form and size in response to its cellular environment. A bacterium can morph into a virus or a fungus cell and back to being a bacterium. These creatures are inside cancer cells. Hulda Clark espoused this theory, as did Dr. Royal Rife, who studied them for many years, and others in the 1930s. (See pp. 9-10 for more on Hulda Clark and pp. 11-13 for more on Dr. Rife.) These pleomorphic microbes can be killed by targeting them with an energy vibration that matches their own. The overdose of energy disintegrates them. Everything on earth is energy and each entity has a vibration rate that can be detected and matched by someone with the right equipment. You may have heard of, or even seen, a soprano singer breaking a wine glass by singing a high note that matches the vibration of the glass energy. That can be done to the microbes in cancer cells and without the microbes, the cells can re-organize themselves and function normally.

4.   A Metabolic Disease

In this context the term "metabolism" refers to all the chemical processes that participate in keeping a cell and its organism alive; that is, **cell** metabolism, not **body** metabolism.

Cancer as a metabolic disease was first articulated by biochemist Otto Warburg in 1924, who found that when oxygen is deficient in body cells, they switch to sugar fermentation. Recent researchers have discovered that all cells generate their energy inside their mitochondria, tiny structures that oxidize glucose. But cancer cells have damaged mitochondria and far fewer of them. So to survive, they ferment glucose instead of oxidizing it, but this is inefficient; it creates far less energy and makes them greedy for more glucose. Their oncogenes get switched on, unleashing uncontrolled cell division. A ketogenic diet keeps glucose very low. The body then uses fats for energy instead of carbohydrates, and instead of producing glucose, the digestive system produces ketone bodies from the breakdown of fats. This all starves the cancer cells.

Assembling Protocol Pieces

Whichever causation theory they espouse, alternative health professionals have devised many and varied protocols They can all be found online and here are some examples:

- **The Budwig Diet Protocol** – used by Dr. Carlos Garcia.* Focuses on getting oxygen into the body cells, enabling them to revert to normal use of oxygen.

- **The Bob Beck Protocol** – Uses microcurrents of electricity to reduce the overall number of pathogens in the body. This lightens the immune system's workload and enables it to focus more on cancer cells.

- **The Bob Wright Protocol** – Based on the infectious disease theory described above; uses organic sulphur, alkkaline water, iodine and other items to kill microbes inside cancer cells, thus reverting the cells to normal use of oxygen instead of glucose.

- **The Kelley Metabolic Protocol** – uses pancreatic enzymes to remove the protective coating on cancer cells, thus enabling the blood's white cells to better identify those cancer cells as undesirables.

Now that I had discontinued the Bill Henderson protocol, I had to decide what alternative to choose. Reading and brooding, I looked back at all the treatments I'd already received and the problems they'd addressed. I kept coming back to acidity and alkalinity, particularly addressed at the Oasis clinic by the raw vegan diet and by the Bill Henderson protocol's plant-based diet.

Perhaps bodily over-acidification contributes to cancer development. Certainly cancer cells thrive in an acidic environment and each of them excretes lactic acid that maintains that environment. (Blood stays at a pH level close to 7.365, slightly alkaline, because the body immediately corrects acidification in blood by drawing calcium from the bones – perhaps this is a cause of brittle bones in older folks. But other fluids can vary a great deal without threatening our life.) Years of acidity in the body's interstitial fluid which surrounds all body cells could be inviting and enabling stray cancer cells to settle in and multiply. Is there any reason why body fluids should be acidic? I haven't come across one. By alkalinizing the body's fluids, we could remove the acidic environment, depriving cancer cells of a home. Evict them.

---

* Dr. Garcia was Bill Henderson's co-author in writing *Cancer Free*. His clinic is in Florida and when Bill Henderson became ill in 2016, he resigned from cancer coaching and went to his friend's clinic. Sadly, he died shortly thereafter at the age of 84, after a hospital attempted a blood transfusion. I was one of his many coachees at that time.

I decided to include alkalinity in my own protocol and add other things I already knew about. To achieve my long-term goal of cancer cure, this protocol would have to:

1. Update some of the testing and re-assemble supplements accordingly;

2. Continue detoxification, keeping the liver and colon clear and freeing the body of any remaining parasites, visible or microscopic;

3. Bring lots of oxygen to all body cells;

4. Be highly nutritious and focus on alkaline food and drinks.

We all need an individual selection of tests so I'll leave that part out here. For the rest, the time at the Oasis of Healing gave me an excellent start. Being in cachexia at that time I'd needed daily IV treatments, frequent non-IV treatments, two blood transfusions, and a platelet pheresis. But I didn't need these any more and everything else done there (e.g. raw vegan diet, veggie juice, wheatgrass, moving the lymph and blood along and clearing the colon), could be continued now at home.

The Bill Henderson protocol could also contribute (Budwig Blend and eliminating parasites and fungus from the gut). So I began putting everything together that I had already used and knew would help and leaving out items I knew or suspected would hinder.

Items to Include

This is my own list; for a more general list of dietary items to include and exclude, see pp. 81-85.

- **All food organic.** Why complicate things by inserting pesticides and herbicides into the body? They kill the beneficial bacteria needed in the gut and create more work for the immune system – as if cancer isn't enough work!

- **Daily Salads.** An obvious item, healthy for everybody, cancer or not.

- **Green Juice**. Every day at Oasis we had as many jars of fresh green juice as we wanted to pay for. I had one 32 oz jar daily. Drinking our vegetables provides the nutrition of many more veggies than we can get by munching them separately. It's highly alkaline also, as are salads.

- **Wheatgrass**. At the Oasis clinic, there had been several big trays of wheatgrass along the bench in a big sunny bow window. When one became ready to use, it was placed next to the special juicer on a nearby table and we could go there any time to make a shot glass of juice. Wheatgrass is loaded with oxygen and a great many other nutrients and is very alkaline.

- **Essiac.** It had successfully dislodged those hordes of worms (p. 177) so best to keep using it. Who knows what else might still be in there?

- **The Budwig Blend.** (pp. 24-25 and p. 85-86) This mixture has been bringing oxygen to body cells since the 1930s as part of Dr. Budwig's anti-cancer diet. It was familiar from my years on the Bill Henderson protocol and is easy to make. It can be enlarged with any mix of veggies, fruit, nuts, and/or seeds to make a complete tasty meal.

- **A vegan diet.** To cancel out the lactic acid produced by cancer cells, this protocol will include an alkalinity based on the raw vegan diet I learned to like at the Oasis clinic.

- **Clean alkaline water**. I resolved to buy a better water filtering system than my jug and to add sodium bicarbonate to the filtered product. This would help alkalinize the body's interstitial fluid.

- **A Trampoline.** It's in a corner of the living room and a daily stint there shakes up the innards and partially compensates for my being unable to dance (since the stroke took some of my balance). Moving the body around daily helps the blood and lymph to move along. The heart pumps the blood faster. Lymph, having no heart, depends on muscle movement to propel it along. If it becomes stagnant, its waste products don't get to the bloodstream and therefore don't get excreted from the body.

Items to Exclude

Sugar. In the cancer context, "sugar" includes honey, agave syrup, coconut nectar, and all other such sweeteners. Xylitol, which I've used since 2012, is remarkable: it doesn't feed cancer, doesn't affect diabetes, doesn't attract ants, doesn't rot the teeth, looks, tastes, and behaves like sugar and has half as many calories. But it is digested down to glucose, as are all carbohydrates: rice, pasta, oatmeal etc.. For a more detailed discussion of the large category of "sugar", see pp. 81-83.

- **Vinegar**. Being an acid, it supports and promotes fungus in the gut. Since I'd been diagnosed in Australia with Candida I decided to avoid anything connected with fungus or mold. So I make salad dressing with lemon or lime juice instead; and no mayonnaise, since it contains vinegar.

- **Mushrooms**. These are a fungus.

- **Tamari and yeast**. Being fermented, they support and promote parasites and since my worm episode I was anxious to make sure the gut was fully clear. I switched to Bragg's Aminos which tastes similar to tamari and is not fermented; and to flat bread like sprouted wheat tortillas and Ezekiel bread that have no yeast.

- **Yogurt and sauerkraut**. These are fermented too. I'd used them for the probiotics but decided to trust my healing gut to take care of that issue.

- **Animal Protein**. All meats and fish are acid-forming when we digest them. We hear often that without meat and/or fish, we'll be lacking in protein but that's not necessarily true. All vegetables and fruits contain some of the 20 amino acids that make up complete protein. The old advice of "Eat lots of vegetables" doesn't mean to pile your plate up high. It means "Eat lots of kinds of vegetables". Another saying is "Eat colorful food"; that is, a wide variety. Following these guidelines, one gets all nine of the essential amino acids and the remaining 11 are made in the body anyway.

Over the past four months, as I've been able, I've now implemented all of the above except Essiac, still to be added.

Benefits So Far

- **The long-time gas-and-constipation problem is solved!** This was a very welcome surprise. Apparently over-acidity had been its cause.

- My eyes don't get tired or dry after about two hours on the computer; they can go for six or seven hours if I have enough sleep.

- The arthritis pain in my fingers has dwindled almost to none. This is partly due to previously starting on collagen powder each day, but I reached a plateau with that. When I started this protocol, the pain reduced even further.

- Assorted chronic itches are gone.

There's much further to go. Hopefully this protocol will work through relatively minor problems and get to the big C quickly. I'll have to be sure I indulge in no lapses or backsliding, but keep up the momentum and get periodic blood tests to see how things are going.

Energy Work #5: Self Protection

An important aspect of doing energy work is protecting yourself from Other People's Energy, OPE. We all throw energy, though we can learn not to, and without any protective measures in place, we are sitting ducks for OPE. When we start to do energy work as adults, we're already full of energy that isn't our own and it has been causing discomfort, confusion and perhaps chronic anger for years. Previous energy work sections have suggested tools for removing that OPE; now let's look at how we can prevent more of it entering our space and interfering with our energy flow. So get comfortable in your energy work chair, check your grounding, and be in the center of your head.

Body of Glass

Think of how light passes through a window – the glass is not changed by sunshine passing through it. We can be that way in regard to OPE. Form the notion that your body and aura are made of glass and will now be unaffected by any OPE that comes your way. Let's say you're getting on the subway and someone throws some anger at you. You're not affected. You don't react and their energy passes right through your body of glass and out the other side and has no effect on your mood or thoughts. Your own energy continues running. If you keep the idea that you're a body of glass, you don't even notice that OPE. It's a non-event. None of it becomes stuck in your space.

Pulling this off requires that you have enough certainty about your own energy to have no guilt about being non-responsive to someone else. You need to be sure in yourself that the integrity of your own energy is more important to you than any person's desire to affect you. Pulling it off also requires that you don't fight the OPE, don't resist it. When we fight something, we involve ourselves with it, become part of it and lose some of our personal freedom. But by keeping the idea of body of glass, we can remain uninvolved and free of OPE.

In other situations, OPE might come at you from someone you care about. This can be a more difficult scenario for self-protection because you have agreements with that person and they know you and how to ruffle you. And you don't want to hurt their feelings or make them feel rejected. Talking to them about doing energy work could help. But some people are control freaks and if they're used to controlling you, they won't take kindly to losing that power. You might have to be firm and teach them that the relationship with you can only stand as long as they stay out of your space.

Protection Rose

Visualize a rose in front of you. Make it any color, blooming or a bud, leaves or not – these things don't matter. Postulate that this rose will intercept all OPE coming at you from any direction. Give it a grounding cord like the one running from your first chakra. This enables it to drain off OPE and keep you free in your own space. From time to time, check on this rose and if it has disappeared, just create another one, the same or different, and ground it.

If you work with a lot of other people, like teaching school or serving in a restaurant, give yourself a fresh protection rose each morning; maybe each lunch time or afternoon; or as often as seems necessary. But even if you work at home, or you're retired and mostly just see friends and family, do yourself the favor of a protection rose. Energy travels through walls and across oceans in an instant: there is no time or space in the energy world.

A Crystal Wall

A third way to protect yourself is what Dr. Büttner suggested to me at the Arcadia Klinik in Germany: put a wall of crystal around your aura with the postulate that OPE cannot penetrate it. I started using this tool and find I like it and it helps me relax more when I'm around strangers. I add a circular grounding cord to the wall so it can drain off whatever OPE hits it. The less OPE we carry around with us, the more free we start to feel and the more like ourselves. It makes for a much happier life.

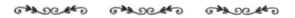

Memorandum

✓ There are four main theories of what causes cancer.

✓ There are many cancer protocols based on the four theories and anyone can choose one to implement.

✓ Gut health is central to general good health and we can all find procedures or products that work for us.

✓ Since cancer cells love an acidic environment, perhaps we can use a vegan diet, fresh vegetable juice, and alkalinized water to make them too uncomfortable to stick around.

✓

✓

✓

Chapter 11: Last But Not Least

Now, as I write this last chapter, it is winter of 2019 and I'm living in southern Illinois to be near my son who has schizophrenia. Although not yet recovered from cancer, I am certainly a cancer survivor, being at eighteen years and counting.

Some Final Thoughts

"In pre-European times in Australia, if an Aboriginal medicine man pointed a bone at one of his tribe, it was a sentence of death. It was a command to go away and die. The recipient of the bone pointing invariably obliged and went away and died. I think there is a lot of this attitude in people who have cancer."

-- *Join Our Escape From Death Row – Cancer Jail,* Barry Thomson, 2007, p. 7. Self published in Australia. He cured his own melanoma that had spread to the lymph system.

A cancer diagnosis is a loud wake-up call, a vigorous tug on your bed covers telling you to get up, get going, nap time is over. It's a bell, either a funeral bell or an alarm bell and you can decide which it is in your case. It means that somehow your immune system has been weakened to the point that it can't cope any more. It's your body calling you,

"Hey, boss! Help! I'm pooped! You gotta take over now so I can rest up and get strong again!"

We are spirits living in physical bodies. These bodies have enormous resilience and can deal with large numbers of poisons for a while, but a cancer diagnosis marks the end of their ability to do so. Unless we get up on our hind legs and take command of our health and our life, we will likely lose the body within months or a few years at most.

This sort of wake-up call does not always take the form of cancer. Many people tumble into a major stroke or a heart attack.

Whether you think you can or think you can't, you're right.

---Henry Ford

It's natural to dislike the idea of changing long-time habits. It's a disruption of the modicum of peace we might feel we've attained, the comfort of knowing what each day will bring, at least to some extent. If we want to survive our cancer diagnosis, we must step back from all this and re-assess how we've been living. The diagnosis tells us that we must take more responsibility for our lives, our health, our daily habits, and even our mental and spiritual health. A well body does not get cancer. There must be established illness, whether officially diagnosed or not, before the body comes down with cancer.

Do Your Homework

For best chances, it's important get informed, to read and research. If you feel too sick or weak to do it yourself, perhaps someone can do it for you. Learn about whatever your conventional doctor is recommending; read about any specific chemo drugs being suggested – their limitations and side effects; about the dangers of radiation treatments; about the risks of surgery. What to do about your cancer is your choice. Doctors may seem persuasive and dominating, but it's your body, your life, and your choice.

At first, the myriad websites on alternative cancer care can be overwhelming but gradually, as with anything new, one gets familiar with the topics and vocabulary. When I started reading about digestion, body chemistry, DNA and related enzymes, how the immune system works, and all the other topics that relate to cancer, I often thought I must be trespassing into the world of some non-human species.

- Twas brillig and the slithy toves did form dehydroepiandrosterone that blocks the leukotriene synthesis from the arachidonic acid cascade and the mome raths outgrabe the shift from TH2 to TH1 through its ethylenediaminetetraacetic acid.[*]

So take advantage of the glossary provided in the next pages. Of course, we patients don't become experienced naturopaths or doctors or knowledgeable microbiologists; but we can learn a great deal from websites and books. Be sure to check out the print and .pdf resource list on pp. 209-211 and the chapter online resources starting on p. 213.

Take Some Time

If anyone is urging you to start chemotherapy NOW, brush him or her aside. Cancer takes months or years to grow to the point of being identifiable by a medical test, so it's not going to strike you down in the next day or two or the next week.

---

[*] Apologies to Lewis Carroll, The Jabberwocky (poem)

Go home and be quiet and think. Ground yourself. Ground off any fear you might have picked up at the doctor's office or elsewhere, and any sense of emergency or hurry. We all feel a bit groggy or slow when we've been rudely woken from our nap and that makes us vulnerable to domination by others.

At a comfortable speed, look around your life circumstances. Something in all your familiar habits, your meals, your comfy home, work routines, relationships, has worked against your health. Probably several things.

I was a slow learner and I don't suggest you take as much time as I did. But I do suggest that you start thinking things through before you submit to any damaging treatment. Part of the job of healing cancer is taking back command of your own life. Own your space. Run your own energy, not your doctor's energy or anyone else's. Make your own decisions. If you have a supportive spouse or relative to help, you're ahead of the game already.

Someone helping – researching for you, making appointments for testing, ordering supplements, keeping the house clean, preparing anti-cancer foods, even just washing the car and filling the tank – gives you immediate practice in feeling gratitude and peace. It will help you relax and release stress, which is part of many people's cancer structure. Over-stressed, over-worked. If you have a job, negotiate for time off work or for working at home.

If you do decide to have chemotherapy, radiation, or surgery, first research how their potentially destructive effects can be mitigated and your immune system supported. You could use Chapter 9, *Offsetting Chemo Harm*, as a starting point.

You might consider forming a support group. Try talking to people in the doctor's waiting room if you're sitting there for a while. Perhaps you know of people in your neighborhood who have cancer or perhaps there are some cancer patients among your friends and family. A support group could be very comforting and encouraging and people could share ideas, recipes, and treatment information and possibly make each other laugh.

And that would be my last thought for you:

- Don't forget to laugh!

Laughing releases stress. That's why people laugh at parties even when they're not really amused. Parties are for fun and no stress. Genuine laughter is a high energy level whereas fear and pessimism are much lower levels; they're "low moods".

We can lift ourselves into higher energy levels if we let go of burdens. Cancer is burden enough, so let go of past worries, old problems, baggage, OPE. People will understand; they know what a demanding thing cancer can be to deal with every day.

> " The pedestrian had no idea which way to go so I ran over him."
>
> "The indirect cause of this accident was a little guy in a small car with a big mouth."
>
> "I had been driving my car for 40 years when I fell asleep at the wheel and had the accident."
>
> "I pulled away from the side of the road, glanced at my mother-in-law, and headed over the embankment."
>
> ---From an insurance company newsletter, early 1990s.

Get into present time and even if things seem grim, or especially when they do, watch a funny movie or read a good joke book or funny novel. Maybe get yourself a kitten or puppy to make you love and laugh. A sense of humor is like a muscle: it develops with use. It might sound bizarre, but you can grow your ability to laugh by laughing when you're not feeling very amused. Perhaps work into it by starting with smiles – smile more often and enjoy the return smiles people will give you. Moving along, laugh at more things; at children's antics, at cats or dogs playing, and feel those laugh muscles working, both physical and emotional. Get them limbered up. You could even just laugh at nothing, though you might want to save this exercise for times when you're alone. ☺

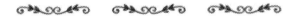

Memorandum

✓ A cancer diagnosis means your body needs help. Go quiet and ask it what it needs from you.

✓ Inform yourself about your cancer and about any treatments being suggested.

✓ Consider starting a support group.

✓ Stay grounded and take time to think about it all so you can make good decisions.

✓ Remember to laugh.

✓

✓

> Zen saying: Spend an hour each day in meditation. Unless you're too busy. In that case, spend two hours.

Glossary

Acetaldehyde	A carcinogen produced in the body by consumption of sugar or alcohol. It damages the DNA.
Adenoids	Lymphatic tissue behind the nasal cavity, part of the immune system.
Adenosine triphosphate	ATP, the body's energy used by all cells and generated in cell mitochondria.
Aerobic	With oxygen.
Agranulocyte	White blood cell containing no granules.
Allergen	A substance that causes an allergic reaction in some people, e.g. gluten, bee pollen, some chemicals.
Amino acid	Building block of proteins.
Amphoteric	Adaptable to either acidic or alkaline environments.
Amylase	A pancreatic enzyme that digests carbohydrates.
Anaerobic	Without oxygen; absence of oxygen.
Angiogenesis	Creation of extra blood vessels to feed a tumor.
Anion	Negatively charged ion, pronounced "an-ion). *cf* Cation
Antibody	A substance created by the body in response to the presence of an antigen.
Antigen	A foreign substance that provokes the immune system to create an antibody to it.
Antioxidants	Molecules that prevent oxidation by donating electrons to free radicals without destabilizing themselves.
Anti-neoplastons	Peptides in the body that inhibit neoplastic (cancerous) cells; name coined by Dr. Stanislav Burzynski, physician and biochemist in Texas who successfully heals cancer patients.
Apoptosis	Cell suicide, performed when a cell becomes damaged or old. Cancer cells perform no apoptosis.

Arachibutyrophobia *	Fear of having peanut butter stick to the roof of your mouth. (a joke to increase your vocabulary)
Artemisinin	Group of drugs that treat malaria; used for cancer.
Artenusate	One of the artemisinin groups of drugs that treat malaria and cancer.
Aspartame	An artificial sweetener that releases aspartate when digested. *Aka* Equal, NutraSweet and Spoonful.
Aspartate	A neurotransmitter used by the brain's neurons. Ingredient of Aspartame. An excitotoxin.
Atom	The smallest unit of matter; consists of a positively charged nucleus with negatively charged electrons around it. All elements on the periodic table are made of atoms. *Cf* ion, molecule.
Autohemotherapy	A cancer treatment where a small amount of blood (100 – 200mls) is removed from the patient, exposed to ultraviolet light, then returned to the patient.
B cells	B Lymphocytes; originate in bone marrow like all blood cells but also mature there (hence the "B"); they differentiate into many types with different functions. *Cf* T cell.
Basal cell carcinoma	One of the three kinds of skin cancer, originating at the deepest level of the skin. *Cf* squamous cell carcinoma and melanoma.
Basophil	A type of granulocyte (white blood cell).
BCR-ABL gene	The faulty compound gene that marks the presence of chronic myeloid leukemia.
Biopsy	Removal of a piece of body tissue for testing.
Blast cell	An immature blood cell normally in the bone marrow until it matures but in myeloid leukemia it enters the bloodstream prematurely.
Blood-brain barrier	A blocking mechanism thought to exist in the walls of capillaries in the brain whereby certain substances are unable to enter brain tissue.

Blood serum	Blood plasma without any clotting elements.
Cachexia	The phase of cancer where one loses weight and appetite from cellular exhaustion. Body cells are unable to make their energy from oxygen and nutrients as they normally do. Because they're exhausted, so is the entire body.
Candida	Overgrowth of Candida albicans, a fungus that is present in everyone's gut but that stays harmless when gut microbes are in balance.
Capillary	Very tiny blood vessel that flows into larger vessels; there are venous capillaries and arterial capillaries.
Carcinogen	Cancer-causing substance.
Carcinoma	Cancer originating in epithelial tissue: the skin and lining of body organs; e.g. basal cell carcinoma originates in the base of the skin's top layer where new skin cells are made. *Cf* sarcoma, melanoma.
Cation	Positively charged ion, pronounced "cat-ion". *cf* Anion.
Cell membrane	The exterior surface of a cell holding many receptors that determine what substances can enter the cell.
Chelation	Removal of heavy metals from the bloodstream, usually via IV; binding agents cause them to be flushed out through feces, urine and sweat.
Chromosome	A two-piece structure that contains a person's DNA (a double helix).
Clonogenic	Tendency to proliferate; potential to generate a colony of identical cells.
Colon hydrotherapy	Use of water to cleanse the colon of accumulated or impacted fecal matter, parasites, undigested food, and mucous.
Cytokines	Signaling molecules that help immune system cells communicate with each other and move towards an injury. (from Greek *cyto* and *kino*s meaning cell and movement) Produced by immune system cells.
Cytotoxic	Poisonous to live cells.

Dialysis	Removal of waste products from the blood when the liver or kidneys are failing or injured.
Digestive enzymes	Enzymes produced by the pancreas and sent to the small intestine to break down food into more absorbable particles.
Digestive system	Mouth, stomach, pancreas, small and large intestines.
Denatured	Of protein: structurally changed; of food or alcohol: deliberately contaminated to make it unfit for consumption while still being suitable for other uses.
Distal to	Anatomical term: distant from the body's median line or a point of origin or attachment. *Cf* proximal to.
Dysbiosis	Imbalance between helpful and harmful bacteria in the gut: overgrowth of harmful bacteria.
Electromagnetic energy	Certain types of radiation, e.g. visible light, radio waves, infrared light, and ultraviolet light.
Endocrine hormone	A powerful hormone (chemical messenger) secreted by an endocrine gland;
Endocrine system	Glands that secrete hormones directly into the bloodstream. There are seven main endocrine glands: pineal and pituitary in the brain; thyroid in the throat; thymus in the chest; adrenal and pancreas in the abdomen; and ovary or testis in the pelvis.
Enzyme	A protein that causes body processes to occur.
Eosinophil	A type of white blood cells known as a granulocyte; it travels to inflamed areas and traps and kills invading organisms such as bacteria or parasites.
Epigenetics	The study of how environmental signals influence gene activity. The environment can be within the body or in the mind and emotions.
Epithelium	The cells that cover both internal and external surfaces of the body. One of the four types of animal tissue with nerve, muscle, and connective tissue.

Erythrocyte	Another name for red blood cell.
Etiology	The cause(s) of a disease; events leading to disease.
Excipient	Inactive ingredient added to a pharmaceutical compound to improve it, e.g. cover a bad taste, increase bulk or lengthen shelf life.
Excitotoxin	A substance that stimulates brain cells. In high enough amounts it kills them.
Extracellular	Outside body cells, e.g. extracellular fluid that keeps the cells moist. It contains interstitial fluid.
Fatty acid	The basic component of a fat or oil.
Free radicals	See Reactive Oxygen Species.
Fluoride	A possible neurotoxin added to public water supplies.
Gastroenterology	Study of the stomach and intestines.
Gene	A segment in a DNA strand; contains instructions for making proteins. We have a copy of each gene from each parent. They exist in each cell's nucleus.
Gene expression	The process by which a gene's instructions are implemented.
Genetically modified (GM or GMO – O for organism)	A chemical company has modified the genes in these plants/crops by merging some with a pesticide so that the plant embodies the pesticide; this saves farmers from spraying. The pesticides cannot be washed off so eating a GM product is eating pesticides, designed to kill microbes and insects. A healthy gut is protected by microbes and if they are killed, gut dysbiosis follows.
Genome	A person's total genetic information, between 30,000 and 50,000 genes.
Genotype	A person's individual combination of genes found in their body cells; their genetic identity.

Gluconeogenesis	The liver's creation of glucose from lactic acid in the blood. A vicious cycle happens where cancer cells incompletely digest glucose, discarding lactic acid into the blood; the liver takes up that lactic acid and converts it back to glucose; the cancer cells ingest that glucose … and so on. Happens during cachexia, starving the body cells and causing the patient to lose weight and muscle strength.
Glutamate	An amino acid used as a neurotransmitter by the brain; in high amounts it becomes an excitotoxin.
Glutamine	Type of amino acid in foods; brain converts it to glutamate for neurotransmission.
Glutathione	Master antioxidant produced by every body cell; central for strong immunity; tends to be low in cancer patients.
Granulation	Formation of grains; also: granulation tissue, the pink tissue that forms around a wound as it heals.
Granules	Enzymes inside the white blood cells known as granulocytes.
Granulocytes	Neutrophils, Eosinophils, and Basophils: white blood cells containing microscopic granules that contain enzymes for digesting microorganisms.
Gut Dysbiosis	Bacterial imbalance in the gut such that harmful microbes outnumber beneficial ones. This opens you to intestinal permeability (leaky gut).
Gyphosate	The active ingredient in Monsanto Corp.'s RoundUp and in many weed killers; highly poisonous to everything living including humans.
Hematopoiesis	Formation of blood cell components from stem cells.
Hemoglobin	The oxygen- and carbon dioxide-carrying protein molecule in red blood cells. It contains iron which helps maintain the cell's shape.

Herxheimer reaction	The body's efforts to quickly lower a high level of toxins through vomiting or diarrhea; also involves nausea and fatigue. Indicates the person overdosed on some form of detoxification.
High density lipoprotein	"Good" cholesterol that keeps blood vessels flexible.
Hodgkin's Lymphoma	A rare type of lymphoma distinguished by the presence of Reed-Sternberg cells.
Hormone	A type of signaling molecule secreted into the blood by endocrine glands; each one travels to certain body areas and makes things happen.
Hydrogenation	Treating a compound or element with hydrogen. Carried out on polyunsaturated oils to keep them solid at room temperatures. Harmful to health.
Hyperbaric oxygen	Pressurized oxygen designed to increase body oxygen levels; delivered in a pressurized chamber.
Hyperthermia	Induced fever; done as a controlled procedure in cancer care to stimulate the immune system.
Hypoglycemia	Low blood sugar.
Hypoxia	Low oxygen level in the body.
Immunoassay	A clinical test to detect specific molecules.
Insulin	A hormone made and secreted by the pancreas in response to the presence of sugar in the blood; it controls blood sugar (glucose) levels.
Insulin Potentiation Therapy	The use of insulin to lower a cancer patient's blood glucose level so that the immediately administered chemotherapy drugs have enhanced power and therefore can be given in low (5% to 10%) doses.
Insulin resistance	A condition where blood sugar level does not respond to insulin so the pancreas produces more and more insulin until it becomes exhausted.

Interleukins	A group of cytokines numbered to identify each; 36 thought to be in the human body though some are fairly unknown. They help regulate immune system responses to infection or inflammation and have functions such as fever induction, growth stimulation and antibody secretion.
Interstitial	Occupying a small area between objects or structures, e.g. interstitial fluid is between body cells. It's part of the body's overall extracellular fluid.
Intestinal Permeability	See Leaky Gut.
Intracellular	Inside a cell, e.g. intracellular fluid.
Ion	Electrically charged atom or group of atoms; can be positively charged (cation) or negatively (anion).
Ionizing radiation	Radioactivity; electromagnetic radiation with enough energy to separate electrons from their atoms or molecules. This turns the atoms or molecules into ions. An example is mammograms, regarded as dangerous because they impose this damage on healthy body cells and can thus be a contributing cause of breast cancer.
Ischemic	Low in oxygen.
IV port	A small device implanted in the upper chest with a narrow tube trailing into a vein. Used for repeated IV treatments.
Ketones	Acidic substances produced in the liver by digestion of fat. When the body hasn't enough glucose or enough insulin, it will start breaking down fat for energy. This can be done for weight loss or as a treatment for cancer. Ketones may also appear in a diabetic person when insulin is too low.
Lactic acid	By-product of a cancer cell's incomplete digestion of glucose.

Leaky gut	A condition of the intestines where necessary bacteria are destroyed by drugs or pesticide-contaminated foods or candida proliferation, so that the gut wall becomes weak. It will develop tiny holes through which food particles pass and enter the blood. Now those particles present to the immune system as foreign bodies that must be captured and excreted. In this way, food allergies (sensitivities) develop.
Leptin	An important hormone produced by fatty tissue; it controls feelings of hunger or fullness. Increases with increased fatty tissue. High leptin levels are usually accompanied by leptin resistance.
Leptin resistance	Inability of the body to respond to leptin's presence; the person does not register messages that the stomach is full and continues eating. Since leptin is a hormone and involved with many body functions, people with leptin resistance cannot lose weight by willing themselves to eat less. However, with help it can be done. Research is ongoing.
Leukemia	Cancer of the blood's white cells originating in the bone marrow.
Leukocytes	White blood cells; there are 6 main kinds: lymphocytes, monocytes, neutrophils, eosinophils, basophils, and macrophages.
Lipase	A pancreatic enzyme that digests fats.
Lipid	A fat or oil.
Low Density Lipoprotein	"Bad cholesterol"; levels can be raised dangerously by eating trans fats, present in most processed foods.
Lymph	A circulating body fluid formed from interstitial fluid; it collects and carries waste substances through lymph vessels and nodes to the venous blood and lacking any pump, depends for propulsion on muscle movement (both smooth and skeletal muscles).

Lymphocyte	A type of white blood cell containing no granules, an agranulocyte. Three kinds: Natural Killer cells, B cells and T cells. More often found in lymph than in blood.
Lymphoid	Resembling lymph; pertaining to lymph. *cf* myeloid.
Lymphoma	Cancer of the lymph system.
Lysing	Disintegration of a body cell by breaking the cell membrane.
Macrophage	A white blood cell, part of the immune system, that chases down invaders, including cancer cells, and engulfs them.
Mast cell	White blood cell similar to basophils but found in tissues rather than blood; helps with wound healing; involved with triggering allergies; the least numerous of the white cells.
Melanoma	Cancer originating in the skin's pigment-forming cells. One of the three types of skin cancer. *Cf* squamous cell carcinoma and basal cell carcinoma.
Melatonin	An endocrine hormone produced by the pineal gland; related to our sleep/wake cycle. Travels in blood to entire body; blood levels rise at night and fall during the day; levels decline with age. Can be taken as a supplement to help with insomnia.
Metabolism	The totality of chemical reactions that happen in an organism to keep it living, i.e. to maintain its energy level. Our energy is produced by individual cells from oxygen and whatever food we eat.
Metabolite	A substance resulting from metabolism.
Metastasis	Spread of cancer cells to other body locations. Also called Seeding. Surgery can cause or spread it through tiny blood drops containing cancer cells getting into healthy tissue.
Methylation	An essential process of life where a methyl group is moved around as part of signaling processes. It needs folate (or choline if insufficient folate), vitamin B6 (pyridoxine) and vitamin B12. A methyl group is a chemical unit made up of 3 hydrogen atoms and a carbon atom.

Microbiome	Gut flora; it consists of beneficial and harmful bacteria and for good health there needs to be a preponderance of beneficial bacteria; otherwise one suffers from gut dysbiosis and the many problems flowing from that.
Microzymas	Name given by Antoine Bechamp (a contemporary of Louis Pasteur) to tiny indestructible entities that he saw as foundational to all life. They exist in all living creatures including humans.
Mitochondria	Tiny structures inside each body cell that produce energy for that cell. The totality of cell energy is the body's energy.
Molecule	Group of two or more atoms with no electrical charge and with a name, e.g. sodium or calcium. *Cf* atom
Monocyte	A type of white blood cell called an agranulocyte that is also a phagocyte as it pursues and engulfs invaders in the blood.
Monounsaturated fat	Oils with a chemical structure that keeps them liquid at room temperature. Examples: olive oil, avocado oil, most nut oils.
Myeloid	Pertaining to bone marrow or the spinal cord. *Cf* lymphoid.
Myeloid stem cell	The progenitor cell that gives rise to the myeloid lineage of blood cells which is all the white cells except lymphocytes.
Natural Killer cells	A type of lymphocyte (white blood cell) Abbrev. NK cells.
Naturopath	A trained health professional who uses herbs, nutrition, massage, and other natural methods and does not use surgery or man-made drugs.
Necrotic	Of body tissue: dead.
Neoangiogenesis	Growth of blood vessels specifically to feed a tumor.
Neoplastic cell	Cancer cell.
Neuron	Electrically excitable nerve cell; sends or receives messages from brain or spinal cord.
Neurotransmitter	Chemical that enables communication between neurons.
Neutrophil	A type of granulocytic white blood cell; it's a first defender against bacteria and fungi. See Granulocyte.

Non-Hodgkin's Lymphoma	Name for a group of cancers of the lymph system involving B cells, T cells and/or NK cells. It can start anywhere in the lymph system and spread to any part of the body.
Oncogene	A gene that can cancerize normal cells and is found in all tumor cells.
Oxidant	An oxidizer, opposite of an antioxidant.
Oxidation	Removal of electrons from a molecule or atom.
Oxidative stress	The total of a body's stress from its normal metabolic creation of free radicals plus environmental sources of oxidation such as toxins in food, water or air. High oxidative stress leads to many diseases, e.g. Parkinson's disease, blood circulation disorders, and cancer.
Oximeter	Small device that fits on a fingertip and reads the pulse rate and the body's oxygen saturation and shows the degree of heartbeat strength.
Ozone	A strongly oxidizing gas formed from oxygen by the addition of a third atom and written as O_3. Has a strong smell that isn't safe to breathe.
Palpate	To examine by touching in diagnosing or assessing the body, e.g. palpate the liver for enlargement.
Pancreas	A gland in the abdomen that belongs in both the endocrine system (makes and secretes insulin) and the digestive system (makes and secretes digestive enzymes).
Partially hydrogenated oils	Trans fats, linked in particular to heart disease and diabetes but used in most processed foods.
Pathogen	A substance, usually a microorganism, that causes disease, e.g. virus, bacteria, fungus. Some scientists hold that these 3 are all forms of the same microbe and this ability to change form is called pleomorphism.
Peptide	Short chain of amino acids, the building blocks of proteins.
Peripheral neuropathy	Nerve damage in the hands, head, or feet that can be caused by chemotherapy.

Ph Chromosome	The hybrid chromosome called BRC-ABL ("BCR Able") that creates dysfunctional white blood cells in chronic myeloid leukemia. Discovered in **P**hiladelphia.
Phagocyte	Type of white blood cell that engulfs and destroys foreign particles in the blood; verb: phagocytose.
Phenotype	The physical expression of a person's genotype: hair color, height, eye color etc.
Pheresis	A procedure that removes blood from a patient or donor, separates it into its main components, removes what is being donated or what is in excess, and returns the rest to the person. e.g. Platelet pheresis removes platelets; leukapheresis removes leukocytes.
PICC line	A catheter inserted in an arm or leg giving IV access to the body; used for repeated treatments to avoid piercing the skin each time. (Peripherally Inserted Central Catheter)
Plasma	The fluid of blood without red, white or platelet cells.
Platelet	Blood cell involved with clotting.
Pleomorphic	Of microbes: able to change themselves from bacteria to viruses to fungi and back again in response to their microscopic environment.
Polyunsaturated fat	Lipid with receptors to hold more hydrogen.
Potentiate	To increase the power (potency) or effectiveness of something e.g. Insulin Potentiation Therapy.
Prostacyclin	A substance made by the body's arteries to help prevent clotting.
Proximal to	Anatomical term: close to the body's median line or to a point of origin or attachment, *Cf* distal to.
Reactive Oxygen Species (ROS)	Free radicals: cells containing oxygen and insufficient electrons; they take electrons from other cells, turning them into free radicals so they in turn take electrons from other cells, … A vicious cycle that damages body tissue.

Redox	A portmanteau word for "oxidation-reduction", referring to cell respiration.
Sarcoma	Cancerous tumor of connective tissue, e.g. bone, fat, or cartilage. *Cf* carcinoma, melanoma
Saturated fat	Lipid with all the hydrogen it can hold.
Septum	Tissue wall that divides other structures from each other, e.g. nasal septum divides the nostrils; interatrial septum divides the heart's two atria.
Slubberdegullion **	A worthless, lazy fellow (17th century).
Spleen	A four-inch organ in the upper left abdomen, behind the rib cage and stomach. Filters old red cells out of the blood, stores a reserve supply of blood, makes antibodies, and stores monocytes until they're needed.
Squamous cell carcinoma	One of the three kinds of skin cancer, originating in the skin's top layer. *Cf* Basal cell carcinoma and melanoma.
Stem cells	Unspecialized cells that can divide themselves and create specialized cells, e.g. skin or stomach cells. Two kinds: embryonic stem cells from fetuses and adult stem cells. Research to date has been done on adult stem cells. We all have our own stem cells.
Substrate	Underlying material; in biochemistry, examples would be a) specific substances on which specific enzymes work; and b) iodine taken as a requirement for the body to make thyroid hormone.
Synergistic	Of groups: working together.
T cells	T lymphocytes; created in bone marrow and developed in the thymus gland (hence the "T"); several kinds with different immune system functions.
Thrombocytes	Another name for blood platelets, clotting cells.
Thrombocytopenia	Low platelet count.

Thymus gland	Endocrine gland in the central chest, active only until puberty when it starts shrinking; part of the immune system, producing hormone Thymosin, necessary for creating T-cells.
Tomography	Display of a three-dimensional image through use of X-rays or ultrasound.
Tonsils	Small masses of tissue at the back of throat, part of lymphatic system.
Trans fat	A partially hydrogenated oil, harmful to heart health; *aka* trans fatty acid.
Triglyceride	Fat compound in body fat; consists of three fatty acids and a glycerol.
Trypsin	Pancreatic enzyme that digests proteins.
Tuberculosis	Infectious bacterial disease, usually affecting the lungs. It can be latent (no symptoms) or active. Antibiotics have been used to treat it and now there are drug-resistant forms of the bacteria. Abbrev. TB.
Twilight anesthesia	Milder dose of surgical anesthesia such that the person is still conscious but feels little or no pain; *aka* conscious sedation.
Tyrosine Kinase	Enzyme that assists in DNA duplication when cells divide. The leukemia drug Sprycel works by inhibiting this enzyme.
Ugsome ***	Loathesome or disgusting (late medieval)
Ultrasound	Sound vibration outside the range of human hearing.
Viscous	Of liquids: thick, gel-like; noun is viscosity.

* and ** and *** Just joking, but it's true. *The Mother Tongue: English and How it Got That Way*, Bill Bryson, William Morrow, 1990, p. 68.

Print and PDF Resources

Many Used in Writing This Saga But Extra Included as Helpful Resources For You

A New Way of Looking at – and Treating – Cancer, Leigh Erin Connealy, M.D., Integrated Health Magazine, Fall Ed., 2014

Budwig Cancer Guide.pdf, www.BudwigCenter.com, Lloyd Jenkins, PhD, ND, EFT (no date provided)

Cancer Free: Your Guide to Gentle, Non-Toxic Healing, Bill Henderson and Carlos M. Garcia, M.D., 4th Ed., 2011

Cancer Research Secrets.pdf: Therapies Which Work and Those Which Don't, Keith Scott-Mumby MD, PhD, Scott-Mumby Author Services, 2nd Ed., 2015, PDF

Diet Wise, Prof Keith Scott-Mumby, MB ChB, MD, PhD, Mother Whale, Inc., 1985, 2005

Dying to be Me, Anita Moorjani, Hay House, 2012

Encyclopedia of Medical Breakthroughs and Forbidden Treatments, Health Secrets and Little-Known Therapies for Specific Health Conditions From A-to-Z, Medical Research Associates, LLC, 2004-13

Excitotoxins: The Taste That Kills, Russell L. Blaylock, M.D., Health Press, Santa Fe, NM, 1997

Fire in the Belly, Keith Scott-Mumby, MD, MB ChB, PhD, Mother Whale, Inc., 2012

Five Levels of Healing, Dietrich Klinghardt, M.D., Ph.D., *Explore*! Vol. 14, Number 4, 2005

Healthy to 100.pdf: An Unconventional Guide to Bullet-Proofing Your Body against Disease, Eliminating Pain, Burning Fat and Living Longer Stronger, Dr. Darrell Wolfe, Wolfe Publishing, 2014

Heal Your Gut With Essential Oils, Dr. Eric L Zielinski, Biblical Health Publishing, 2016

Healing Cancer With Common Sense, Marcus and Sabrina Freudenmann, self-published in Australia, 2012.

Living Foods for Optimum Health, Brian R. Clement with Theresa Foy DiGeronimo, Three Rivers Press, 1998

Medical Medium, Anthony William, Hay House, Inc., 2015

My Stroke of Insight, Jill Bolte Taylor, Ph.D., Penguin Group, 2006

Nature's First Law: The Raw-Food Diet, Arlin, Dini & Wolfe, Maul Brothers Publishing, 2003

Nature's Number One Healing Secret.pdf, Keith Scott-Mumby, MD, MB ChB, PhD (no date provided)

One Man's Life-Changing Diagnosis: Navigating the Realities of Prostate Cancer, Craig T. Pynn, DemosHEALTH, 2012

Outsmart Your Cancer, Tanya Harter Pierce, M.A., MFCC, ThoughtWorks Publishing, 2nd Ed., 2009

Rainbow Green Live Food Cuisine, Gabriel Cousens, M.D. and Tree of Life Café Chefs, North Atlantic Books, 2003

Salvestrols: Nature's Defense Against Cancer, Brian A. Schaefer, Clinical Intelligence Corp., 2012

Shopper's Guide to Pesticides in Produce.pdf, Environmental Working Group, 2015 (List of their Dirty Dozen and Clean Fifteen)

Sick and Tired?, Reclaim Your Inner Terrain, Robert O. Young, Ph.D., D.Sc. with Shelley Redford Young, L.M.T., Woodland Publishing, 2001

Side Effects: Death, John Virapen, 2nd Ed., Money Tree Publishing, 2015

Taking the Mystery Out of Cancer.pdf, Dr. David W. Tanton, Ph.D., Soaring Heights Publishing, 2011

The 31-Day Home Cancer Cure, Ty Bollinger with Andrew Scholberg, Online Publishing and Marketing, L.L.C., 2012

The Biology of Belief, Bruce H. Lipton, Ph.D., Hay House, 2008

The Budwig Cancer and Coronary Heart Disease Prevention Diet, The Complete Recipes, Updated Research & Protocols for Health & Healing, Dr. Johanna Budwig, Freedom Press, 2011. (Introduction by Bruce Barlean of Barlean's Organic Oils, who personally knew and learned from Dr. Budwig.)

The Coconut Oil Miracle, Bruce Fife, C.N., N.D., Penguin Group, 2004

The Cure to Cancer Book: 27 Experts Share New Research and Insights on Integrative Approaches to Preventing, Healing, and Reversing Cancer, Hosted by Jean Swann, Panacea Publishing, 2014

The Detox Solution, Dr. Patricia Fitzgerald, Illumination Press, 2000

The Emotion Code: How to Release Your Trapped Emotions for Abundant Health, Love, and Happiness, Dr. Bradley Nelson, Wellness Unmasked Publishing, Mesquite, NV, 2007

The Transformational Power of Fasting, Stephen Harrod Buhner, Healing Arts Press, 2012

Toxic Food Syndrome, Jeffrey S. Zavik & Jim Thompson, Fun Publishing, 2002

Tripping Over the Truth, Travis Christofferson, CreateSpace Independent Publishing Platform, 2014

You Gotta Have Guts! The Natural Way to Enhance G.I. Health, Victoria Bowmann, pH.D., Bow-Mac, Inc., 2009

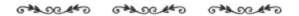

Online Resources Per Chapter

General

http://medical-dictionary.thefreedictionary.com/

http://www.innerbody.com/ Interactive anatomy site

http://www.healthline.com/human-body-maps/ Interactive anatomy site, excellent IMO

https://www.boundless.com/physiology/textbooks/boundless-anatomy-and-physiology-textbook/blood-17/ A well-organized collection of anatomy and physiology lessons

http://www.cancertutor.com/ Large and informative site

http://drleonardcoldwell.com/ Large site with material on many health-related topics

https://www.boundless.com/physiology/ comprehensive site on physiology

http://www.ewg.org/ Environmental Working Group ; a very extensive and detailed site

http://www.ewg.org/skindeep/ Information on personal care products

http://www.utopiawellness.com/services/alternative-cancer/ Overview of a holistic approach to cancer

https://healthy-living.org/ Many health-improvement products with exceptionally clear and detailed text on how each one works.

http://doctorsaredangerous.com/ Large site on many health and cancer topics

http://globocan.iarc.fr/Pages/Map.aspx Interactive world map of cancers; click on "world", "incidence" etc. to get drop-down menus.

https://thetruthaboutcancer.com/ Ty Bollinger has interviewed cancer-wise people worldwide and gives tons of valuable information.

https://www.holisticprimarycare.net/blog/roby-mitchell-blog/1292-infection-or-overgrowth-.html Explains the differences between infections and overgrowths and how each should be treated.

http://cancerremedies.net/burzunsky-cancer-cure-finally-released-by-the-feds/ Dr. Burzynski in Dallas, TX, won another court case against the federal government and Big Pharma

www.cancerdefeatedpublications.com Sells recent books about cancer treatments and offers a newsletter about such treatments

http://www.anoasisofhealing.com/alternative-cancer-treatments-do-they-work/ Article by Dr. Thomas Lodi, founder and director of An Oasis of Healing

https://ghr.nlm.nih.gov/handbook/howgeneswork?show=all Clear and succinct site on genes and proteins

http://www.naturalnews.com/027020_cancer_AMA_treatment.html A large news site on natural healthcare; this page gives the story of Harry Hoxsey who cured cancer with a mix of herbs used by Native Americans, along with a skin salve and a specific diet. His clinics were shut down but he opened another one in Tijuana that is still operating.

http://www.voxnature.com/how-he-cured-himself-of-leukemia-without-drugs-or-radiation/ A diabetic man cured his own Chronic Lymphocytic Leukemia and improved his blood sugar levels in the process.

Introduction

http://www.huffingtonpost.com/2013/12/17/glaxosmithkline-pay-doctors_n_4457286.html In 2014 this pharmaceutical company announced cessation of payments to doctors for promoting the company's drugs

http://www.wsj.com/articles/glaxosmithkline-found-guilty-of-bribery-in-china-1411114817 In 2012, this company was handed a huge fine

Chapter 1: Diagnosis

http://www.chrisbeatcancer.com/what-every-new-cancer-patient-needs-to-know/ The four pro-cancerous conditions

http://www.beating-cancer-gently.com/ Bill Henderson's website; you can buy his book and sign up for his newsletter. Bill Henderson died in 2016 but his wife is continuing his newsletter

http://www.lifeone.org/AMAS_TEST.html A blood test to diagnose cancer. Site gives information and instructions. FDA-approved and covered by Medicare.

http://www.cancertutor.com/ A detailed and comprehensive site for all stages and types of cancer; offers excellent basic education and information on many successful protocols.

https://www.webmd.com/heart/anatomy-picture-of-blood#2 A summary site on blood conditions and tests.

http://www.drclark.net/ Comprehensive information on Hulda Clark

http://rifedigital.com/dr-royal-rife-discovers-the-cure-for-cancer/ A comprehensive site on Dr. Rife's life and work.

http://rifevideos.com/rife_machine_technology.html Information on Rife's machines and his discoveries and achievements in regard to cancer

https://archive.org/details/RoyalRaymondRife 2 hour video on Rife's microscope

NOTE: There are many websites for people freshly diagnosed with cancer that I don't list here because their text is based on the assumptions that (1) you're going to die pretty soon; and 2) you have only a conventional cancer doctor. Depending on your situation, some sites might be helpful to some extent but I would caution you not to get enmeshed in their often subtle negativity.

Chapter 2: A Wake-up Call

https://thetruthaboutcancer.com/bill-henderson-cancer-tribute/ A website on cancer with a tribute to Bill Henderson, who died in 2016

https://budwigcenter.com/ A Budwig clinic

https://gerson.org/gerpress/the-gerson-therapy/ The Gerson Institute in San Diego

https://www.anoasisofhealing.com/ A non-residential cancer clinic that offers a full range of immune-boosting and cancer-killing treatments and provides three good raw vegan meals per day.

http://dayspringcancerclinic.com/ A non-residential cancer clinic in Scottsdale, AZ that offers a very wide range of alternative treatments.

Chapter 3: Emergency IV Care

http://cancerimmunotherapycentres.com/ipt.php A detailed page on what Insulin Potentiation Therapy is and what it is not

https://riordanclinic.org/what-we-do/high-dose-iv-vitamin-c/ Benefits of IV vitamin C

http://www.lifeworkswellnesscenter.com/cancer/ozone-therapy-for-cancer.html How ozone and oxygen help a cancer patient

http://www.utopiawellness.com/services/chelation-therapy/ How EDTA clears toxins and heavy metals from the body

http://www.cancercenterforhealing.com/cancer-treatments/autohemotherapy/ The many ways that ultraviolet light improves health

Chapter 4: Non-IV Treatment

http://www.drlwilson.com/articles/COFFEE%20ENEMA.HTM#CH1 comprehensive information on coffee enemas

http://www.drlwilson.com/articles/PEYER'S%20PATCHES.htm Much information on the Peyer Patches, part of the immune system.

http://www.vivo.colostate.edu/hbooks/pathphys/digestion/basics/index.html A good and complete overview of the digestion system

http://www.myrealhealth.com/index Site of Victoria Bowmann, author of *You Gotta Have Guts!* (see Print & PDF Resources). Sells many products for intestinal health.

http://www.cancercenterforhealing.com/cancer-treatments/lymphatic-therapy/ Good information on lymph and how its flow can be improved

https://summitsucess.wordpress.com/2013/11/13/how-does-the-lymphatic-system-work/

http://cancercompassalternateroute.com/ Large collection of pithy and informative articles related to cancer and health improvement

https://hippocratesinst.org/colon-hydrotherapy-2 A fairly long list of FAQs on colon hydrotherapy

https://pulsedenergytech.com/pemf/ A brief history of PEMF from 2,000 BC to now.

Chapter 5: A Diet to Discourage Cancer

http://www.fda.gov/ForConsumers/ConsumerUpdates/ucm372915.htm

Announcement that trans fats must be listed on food labels

http://www.fda.gov/Food/IngredientsPackagingLabeling/FoodAdditivesIngredients/ucm079609.htm FDA explaining trans fats

http://www.ewg.org/research/ewg-s-dirty-dozen-guide-food-additives

http://www.foodnews.org/ 9 links to downloadable shopping guides, e.g. "EWG's Shopper's Guide to Pesticides in Produce" and "EWG's Guide to Healthy Cleaning"; and other links to related information

http://www.thehealthsite.com/diseases-conditions/reasons-junk-foods-are-bad-for-your-health-sh214/ 10 bad things re junk food; Clear; large health site;

http://tinyurl.com/jobfqsq Dr. Mercola on what happens when we eat junk food; video of stomach;

http://www.healthyvitaminsrx.com/ Much information on vitamins and some other topics

http://draxe.com/ Large site on countless health and nutrition topics

http://articles.mercola.com/omega-3.aspx Get a balance of 3 and 6; sources;

http://tinyurl.com/jsgffa6 Dr. Mercola's analysis of chocolate and its nutritional content;

https://www.betterhealth.vic.gov.au/health/conditionsandtreatments/pancreas Pancreas info;

http://doctoryourself.com/cancer_2.html Nutritional suggestions for cancer treatment;

http://tinyurl.com/haa9j8k FDA definitions of label terms;

http://healthwyze.org/reports/190-the-true-budwig-protocol Gives details of the complete Budwig protocol and a lot of good advice;

http://phmiracleliving.com/t-food-chart.aspx Detailed lists of acid and alkaline foods;

http://articles.mercola.com/sites/articles/archive/2009/08/18/the-secrets-of-resveratrols-health-benefits.aspx Resveratrol information;

http://www.nutrition-and-you.com/coconut-water.html

http://coconutoil.com/virgin-coconut-oil-for-skin-health/ testimonials;

http://tinyurl.com/h7vrys6 Dr. Mercola: information on sugar, artificial sweeteners, trans fats and vitamin D;

http://www.livestrong.com/article/556918-the-disadvantages-of-erythritol/ Information on erythritol;

http://tinyurl.com/zs745b4 An Oasis of Healing: Description of green juice ingredients and why they're used to treat cancer;

Chapter 6: Stem Cell Treatments in Thailand

http://www.ncbi.nlm.nih.gov/pmc/articles/PMC3757281/ Research article finding that papaya leaf does raise red cell and platelet counts

http://www.top10homeremedies.com/how-to/increase-low-platelet-count.html Papaya leaf tea, some vegetables and other ways

https://www.cellmedicine.com/types-of-stem-cells/ Clear information on umbilical cord stem cells and adult stem cells and on treatments using your own.

http://www.closerlookatstemcells.org/learn-about-stem-cells/ Informative site, good basic information, a page on nine things to be cautious about.

Chapter 7: Getting Some Testing

http://www.navarromedicalclinic.com/ A urine test of the presence of cancer cells even before "signs or symptoms develop". Good way to gauge your progress on a protocol. Complete instructions. Done in the Philippines.

http://www.liver.ca/liver-health/ Good summary of liver health and liver disease

http://www.endocrineweb.com/conditions/hyperthyroidism/hyperthyroidism-overview-overactive-thyroid Information on hyperthyroidism

https://www.genome.gov/27530687 Explains biological pathways

http://www.lifeone.org/AMAS_TEST.html A blood test to diagnose cancer. Site gives information and instructions. FDA-approved and covered by Medicare.

http://www.euro-med.us/dr-kobayashi-story.pdf Article on Tsuneo Kobayashi, a Japanese doctor and biochemistry researcher who has developed the ONCOblot blood test that detects cancer years before any conventional test can.

http://oncoblotlabs.com/ Site offering a brochure about this test and information on how to get tested. It confirms the presence or absence of 25+ cancers including leukemia.

http://www.oncolabinc.com/ Related site offering the AMAS test, an older and some say less reliable test than ONCOblot.

http://vitaminmineraltest.com/ Nutritional testing that does not require a doctor's order; test kits supplied, help given in finding a lab for a blood draw. (It appears to be shut down now.)

http://www.walkinlab.com/vitamin-and-nutrition-tests.html Offers a wide variety of testing such as liver function, allergies, hormones and digestive system. Many discounted prices.

https://www.spectracell.com/ Has a clinician side and a patient side; offers comprehensive micronutrient testing.

Chapter 8: Hyperthermia in Germany

http://www.arcadia-cancer-treatment.com/arcadia-cancertreatment/treatments/hyperthermia/ldh/ Local hyperthermia, how it works

http://www.arcadia-cancer-treatment.com/arcadia-cancertreatment/treatments/hyperthermia/wbh/ Whole body hyperthermia; explains what fever is and why we should not rush to reduce it

https://www.anoasisofhealing.com/iv-vitamin-c-for-cancer-treatment/?inf_contact_key=7a77aea3985a6faa33848737149195a7 Explains why oral vitamin C can't do what high dose IV vitamin C can do

http://www.thedcasite.com/dca_how_it_works.html Much information on DCA (dichloroacetate) and how it works to kill cancer cells

https://www.drpawluk.com/education/ Information on magnetic field therapy; the difference between PEMF and EMF and how PEMF is healing

http://yaletownnaturopathic.com/how-does-artesunate-kill-cancer/

http://www.cancure.org/12-links-page/43-artemesia How artemisia (wormwood) works to kill cancer cells

Chapter 9: Offsetting Chemo Harm

http://www.chrisbeatcancer.com/why-i-didnt-do-chemo/ Chris Wark's reasons for his decision

http://www.mayoclinic.org/tests-procedures/chemotherapy/basics/how-you-prepare/prc-20023578

http://www.cancure.org/12-links-page/91-dealing-with-the-side-effects-of-chemotherapy-and-radiation Many practical tips on reducing chemo harm

http://www.naturalnews.com/050540_chemotherapy_nerve_gas_chemicals_Dr_Nicholas_Gonzalez.html Video interview with Dr. Nicholas Gonzalez about how chemo drugs were first developed; also text on his background.

http://www.utopiawellness.com/services/rebuild-after-chemo/ An out-patient program for restoring your health after chemotherapy

Chapter 10: A New Protocol

https://www.anoasisofhealing.com/

https://www.arcadia-praxisklinik.de/

https://www.scienceabc.com/humans/what-is-the-ideal-ph-of-the-body.html

https://www.thealternativedaily.com/signs-your-body-is-too-acidic/

https://www.healthline.com/nutrition/wheatgrass-benefits

https://www.healthline.com/nutrition/wheatgrass-benefits#section3

https://www.askdrsears.com/topics/feeding-eating/family-nutrition/vegetables/7-reasons-why-veggies-are-so-good-for-you

http://ga2.mylifeline.org/ A non-profit that provides free websites for cancer patients so you can keep friends and family informed, post blogs, raise funds, and much else.

https://cancerfightingstrategies.com/ph-and-cancer.html Large site with clear explanatory text. I know nothing about the supplements they recommend.

https://www.canceradvocacy.org/cancer-advocacy/survivor-stories/ This site is "inside the box" and you can read about the appalling treatment misery people went through yet emerged as double survivors – from the treatments and the disease.

http://www.canceractive.com/cancer-active-page-link.aspx?n=3430&Title=Fiona%20beat%20cancer%20twice,%20leukaemia%20and%20ovarian%20cancer A heartening story; she used the Gerson Therapy, IPT (see p. 42) and hyperthermia (see p. 152) among other things and she did energy work. This site has many survivor stories.

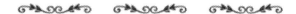

About the Author

Jen Kimberley was born and raised in Australia and came to America in 1963 as a music student. She graduated with a Masters in music, married, obtained a green card, and had two sons. Later, she became an American citizen and thus has dual citizenship. She has mostly worked as a writer, first for technical manuals and then for websites.

Her cancer diagnosis was in November 2001 so as of this date, November 2019, she is eight years past the nine to ten years officially allotted to her by the medical establishment. Her cancer treatments, after eight years of a leukemia chemo pill, have been provided by alternative cancer clinics in Arizona and Germany. She also spent a year or so in Thailand getting two stem cell treatments.

Despite all this and her organic, anti-cancer diet with many supplements, she still tests positive for Chronic Myeloid Leukemia. She has devised a new protocol that is covered in Chapter 10. Her website at www.jenkimberley.com will document her progress on it and discuss many health- and cancer-related topics. On that site you can sign up to be on her mailing list.

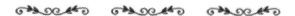

Index

Printed in the United States
By Bookmasters